Midwives and Medical Men

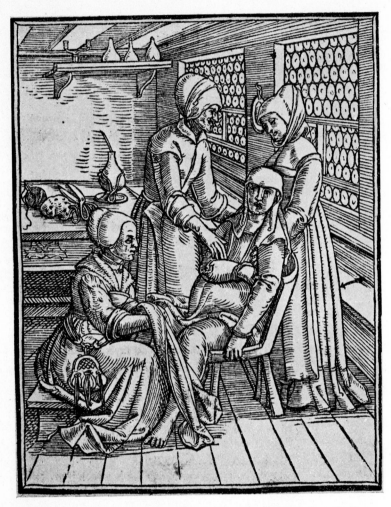

Midwife attending childbearing woman seated on obstetrical stool. From Jacobus Rueff *Ein Schön Lnstig Trostbüchle von den Empfengknussen und Geburten der Menschen*, Zurich, 1554, by courtesy of the Wellcome Trustees.

MIDWIVES AND MEDICAL MEN

A History of Inter-Professional Rivalries and
Women's Rights

JEAN DONNISON

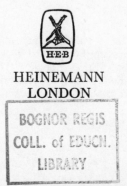

HEINEMANN
LONDON

Heinemann Educational Books Ltd
LONDON EDINBURGH MELBOURNE AUCKLAND TORONTO
HONG KONG SINGAPORE KUALA LUMPUR NEW DELHI
NAIROBI JOHANNESBURG LUSAKA IBADAN
KINGSTON

ISBN 0 435 32250 8

Published by
Heinemann Educational Books Ltd
48 Charles Street, London W1X 8AH
Printed and bound in Great Britain by
Morrison & Gibb Ltd, London and Edinburgh

Contents

Index to Plates

Acknowledgments

In writing this book I have had generous help from many people. In particular, I wish to thank Professor Brian Abel-Smith of the London School of Economics and Political Science, who supervised my thesis, *The Development of the Profession of Midwife in England, 1750–1902*, on which all but the final chapter is based, and Professor O. R. MacGregor of Bedford College, for reading the thesis manuscript and making some valuable suggestions.

I owe a special debt of gratitude to Mr. J. L. Thornton, Librarian of the Medical School at St. Bartholomew's Hospital, for his kind encouragement and assistance at the beginning of my enquiries. Since that time there have been many librarians and archivists who have given me generously of their time and knowledge. Chief among these were the staff of the British Museum Library, the Bodleian Library, the Fawcett Library, the Guildhall Library, the Library of the Society of Friends, the Library of the Royal College of Physicians, the Library of the Royal College of Surgeons, the Library of the Royal College of Obstetricians and Gynaecologists, the Library of the Royal College of Nursing, the Lambeth Palace Library, the Public Record Office, the Greater London Record Office (in particular, Miss Joan Kenealy), the Queen's Nursing Institute, and the staff of the Wellcome Institute Library, on whose inexhaustible patience I came to depend so largely.

I want to thank the Royal College of Midwives, whose kindness and tolerance were invaluable to me during the early stages of my research, also the Royal College of Physicians, the Royal College of Surgeons, the British Hospital for Mothers and Babies, Woolwich, Queen Charlotte's Maternity Hospital, the City of London Maternity Hospital, the Liverpool Maternity Hospital, St. Mary's Hospital, Manchester, the Jessop Hospital for Women, Sheffield, and the Society of Medical Officers of Health (now the Society of Community Medicine) for making available to me the unpublished records of their respective institutions. Without their help my research would not have been possible.

I am also grateful to Jean L'Esperance, Brenda Sutton, Heidi Olsen and Rachel and Polly Donnison for their help in the final preparation of my manuscript, to Mary Bishop for her patient care in typing it, and to my son Christopher Donnison for the many journeys he made to take it to her.

CHAPTER ONE

The Office of Midwife

The office of midwife is an ancient one. From time immemorial women have helped each other in childbirth, and midwives have been recorded from the beginning of history. Midwives appear in Genesis, and in Exodus two midwives, Shiprah and Puah, are rewarded by God for their part in outwitting Pharaoh. In the ancient world childbirth was regarded as a female 'mystery' of which women alone had special knowledge and understanding, and which was presided over by female deities, like Isis, Juno Lucina, and Diana, to whom pregnant women prayed for safe deliverance in their travail. Hence, until comparatively recent times, the work of attending childbirth remained 'women's business'. Moreover, in accordance with the old principle that experience is the best teacher, tradition required that only women who had themselves borne children should perform this office.

This is not to say that male physicians never interested themselves in midwifery. Hippocrates, Aristotle, Celsus, Galen, and other writers on medical matters devoted part of their works to the subject, and the career of Soranus of Ephesus, an outstanding obstetrician and gynaecologist who flourished in Rome in the early second century A.D., shows that by this time some men were actually practising it. However, Soranus' writings make it clear that the work was generally undertaken by women. Although in his *Fables* the Roman writer Hyginus tells us that the ancient Athenians once forbade the practice of midwifery and medicine to women and slaves,[1] this story is uncorroborated, and is probably apocryphal.

But women did not confine themselves to the practice of midwifery alone. Traditionally, they had always cultivated the healing arts. Not only did the treatment of the diseases of their sex naturally fall to them, but there were many women who also practised general medicine, and who, like the celebrated Aspasia, the second-century Graeco-Roman surgeon and obstetrician, achieved a wider distinction as physicians and surgeons. This tradition continued in

I

mediaeval Europe, including England. The practice of medicine and surgery was commonly undertaken by nuns of the local convent, or by the lady of the manor, as part of a charitable duty. But there were also women who practised for money. These ranged from the educated woman like Cecilia of Oxford, employed as Court surgeon by Queen Philippa, wife of Edward III, to the 'wise women' of the village whose remedies would be a compound of common sense, experience and the superstition which formed part of mediaeval medical practice even at the most exalted levels.

Until the thirteenth century practice in the whole field of medicine appears to have been open to all, men and women, whether possessed of education and training or not. The only distinction available to the better educated man was the Licence granted to graduates in medicine by the Universities of Oxford and Cambridge, which conferred the right to practise throughout the whole country under the title of 'Physician' or 'Doctor'. Women were barred from the Universities, however, and in consequence this official recognition of medical skill and status was not available to the female practitioner.

With the thirteenth century came the development of the barber-surgeons' guilds, and with them the regulation of surgical practice in those towns where the guild system was in force. The guild laid down conditions for apprenticeship and admission to membership and undertook the oversight of practice among its members. In return for its part in guaranteeing standards of practice, the guild's members were granted exclusive rights within the town and its environs, and the privilege of prosecuting those engaging in this work without the guild's licence. Women were occasionally admitted to membership, either by apprenticeship or patrimony, but their number does not seem to have been large.

The development of surgeons' guilds was to have an important effect on the work of midwives, since under the guild system the right to use surgical instruments belonged officially only to the surgeon. The surgeon was therefore considered the appropriate person to send for in labours where natural delivery was not possible. All he could do, however, before the invention of the midwifery forceps in the seventeenth century, was to remove the infant piece-meal by use of hooks and perforators, or, if there was still hope of delivering a living child, to perform a Caesarian section on the body of the mother after her death. Since he was called in to abnormal cases only, the surgeon had little opportunity of gaining a real understanding of the process of parturition, and his advent in the lying-in room presaged the death of mother or child, if not both.[2]

In the absence of a surgeon, the midwife herself might perform such an operation and, in the event of the mother's death, she had a duty laid on her by the Church to extract the child by Caesarean section in order that it should not die unchristened and its soul be lost. Thus a fifteenth-century manual outlining the duties of the parish priest advises him:

> And ȝef the wommon thenne dye,
> Teche the mydwyf that scho hye
> For to undo hyre wyth a knyf
> And for to save the chyldes lyf
> And hye that hyt crystened be,
> For that ys a dede of charyte.[3]

Not much is known about English midwives in the Middle Ages. It is likely that they were married women, of middle age or older, who had themselves borne children; indeed, right to the end of the seventeenth century personal experience of childbirth was still generally regarded as an essential qualification.[4] Maturity itself was also considered an advantage. An older woman might herself have gone through childbirth many times. She would also have seen many of her neighbours give birth, since the tradition in all social classes was to summon friends and relations who had themselves borne children to witness the proceedings.[5]

This custom fulfilled several needs. First, the presence of a number of experienced women could provide support to the mother during a trying and possibly dangerous ordeal. Second, in enabling older women to acquire greater knowledge of the processes of childbirth such gatherings clearly had an important educative function, of especial significance to the large part of the population unable to obtain the services of a formally trained or 'professed' midwife. Third, these gatherings ensured that there were witnesses to the birth. If the child did not live, the testimony of these women could protect the mother from suspicions that she herself had caused its death. Conversely, their presence could prevent the substitution of children in cases where the mother, desperate to escape the stigma of childlessness or of failure to produce a male heir, might attempt to pass off as her own the child of another.[6] Finally, in a society where life was often hard, they provided a welcome occasion for a neighbourly celebration.

Maturity in the midwife may also have been important to the Church, which in mediaeval and post-Renaissance Europe wielded great power over people's day-to-day lives. Church Courts exercised jurisdiction in a wide range of human affairs, including matters which now fall within the area of private morality. Hence the midwife's character and religious beliefs were of vital concern to the ecclesiastical authorities who were anxious that she should not shield from discovery and punishment those falling short of the standards of chastity laid down by the Church. She was therefore expressly forbidden to perform any act leading to the destruction of the child or the concealment of the birth, though then, as later, the production of abortions was an activity not limited to women.[7] She also had to do her best to make the mother of a bastard infant name the father, in order that he might not evade his duty to maintain his offspring, nor escape the punishment that could be inflicted for his offence in fathering it.

Again, it was part of Christian doctrine that the soul of a baby which died unbaptized would lose its chance of salvation; hence it was the midwife's duty to baptize any child thought likely to die before it could be taken to the priest. Moreover, it was vital that this be done according to the approved form, and a midwife who used the wrong words, and so 'lost a chylde, bothe soule and lyfe', was commanded by the priest that

> . . . she shulde no more
> Come eftesones where chyldryn were bore.[8]

Indeed, the whole process of childbirth was the focus of a mass of ancient superstitious beliefs which still played an important part in Christian thinking. The act of giving birth was believed to defile the mother, who could be re-admitted to the Church only after a service of purification or 'churching'. Moreover, the fact that the umbilical cord, caul, afterbirth and still-born foetus played an important part in the rites of witchcraft provided additional justification for the Church's attempts to control midwives and to punish those who in any way departed from the prescribed code.

The Rolls of York Minster record such a prosecution. In 1481 Agnes Marshall of Emeswell in Yorkshire was 'presented' before the Bishop's Court, not merely because she lacked experience and skill, but because she also used incantations.[9] On the Continent, where the fear of witchcraft was stronger, midwives were at greater risk. In Paris in 1409 the midwife Perrette was 'turned' in the pillory and banned from practice for (unwittingly) supplying a foetus for use in magical rites.[10] *The Hammer of the Witches* (1484–6), the classic work on witchcraft by Sprenger and Institoris, two German members of the Inquisition, warned that no-one did more harm to the Catholic faith than midwives, who 'surpass all other witches in their crimes'. Witch-midwives, it was claimed, often killed the infant they were delivering, either at the birth, or while it was yet in the womb, dedicating its soul to their master, the devil, and in Germany at this time women were actually executed on such charges.[11] In some states midwives had to report the birth of monsters, which were thought to be the devil's offspring, and if the mother had not led a manifestly blameless life, she herself stood in great risk of being accused as a witch.[12]

But by the middle of the fifteenth century the regulation of midwives on the Continent was no longer being left solely to the Church. Many cities in Germany and the Netherlands already showed active concern for the health of their people, appointing City Physicians with the duty of controlling medical practice and attending the poor. In 1452 the city of Regensburg went a step further, instituting what is believed to have been the first municipal system of midwife regulation in Europe, an example which was to be widely followed within the next hundred years. Some cities also appointed midwives to serve the poor, and in Regensburg itself there was provision for aged and disabled midwives to be relieved from the town coffers.[13]

Under municipal regulation midwives were still required to show evidence of good character, bind themselves not to procure abortions, and so on, nor practise any magical rites. But more attention was paid by the municipal authorities than by the Church to questions of technical competence. Midwives setting up on their own account were formally examined on this point, either by a physician (who, however, probably derived what knowledge he had of the subject from ancient texts, rather than actual practice) or by experienced midwives appointed for the purpose.[14] In Paris, where this system also applied, the examination was the duty of a panel of surgeons and midwives acting together. However, these systems of municipal regulation also had the effect of limiting the scope of the midwife's practice. Most of them required her to send for the assistance of a doctor or surgeon in difficult births, and in Strasbourg she was prohibited from using hooks or other sharp instruments on pain of death.[15]

In England the first formal arrangements for the control of midwives were made under an Act of 1512. In line with the general Tudor policy of strengthening the control of central government, the Act aimed at securing the nation-wide regulation of medicine and surgery. According to the Act's preamble, many practitioners in these fields were merely 'common artificers, as smithes, weavers, and women', who not only lacked appropriate skills for their work, but also employed witchcraft[16] to aid their cures. It therefore provided for a system of licensing skilled and approved practitioners, and for the punishment or suppression of the rest.

Responsibility for the implementation of the Act was laid on the ecclesiastical authorities. The Church already had a direct interest in eliminating witchcraft; it was also the only authority with the machinery necessary for the Act's enforcement in country districts. All persons seeking a licence, therefore, with the exception of graduates licensed by the Universities, were required to submit themselves for examination by the local Bishop. He was empowered to seek expert testimony on the candidate's suitability, and, if satisfied, to grant a licence for independent practice in the diocese. Persons practising without a licence were liable to be 'presented' at the Bishop's Court and punished.

Though the Act did not mention midwives, they were licensed under its provisions soon afterwards, probably on the basis that midwifery was considered a part of surgery. Anxiety about the use of 'sorceries and witchcrafte' in medicine had been one of the justifications for the Act, and it was only logical that the Church should seize this opportunity more effectively to prevent its practice in connection with childbirth. Midwives were therefore also required to apply to the Bishop's Court, and if granted a licence, to take a solemn oath swearing to obey the rules of conduct which the Church laid down for their practice.

The oath was long and detailed. In the diocese of Canterbury in 1567 Eleanor Pead promised to 'faithfully and diligently exercise the said office' (of midwife) 'according to such cunning and knowledge as God hath given me', and to be ready to assist 'as well poor as rich'. She also swore that she would not use 'any kind of sorcerie or incantation in the time of travail of any woman', and that when called on to christen a child she would baptize it with plain water only, using the 'apt and accustomed' form, and 'none other profane words'. Other provisions of her oath were directed at preventing the false attribution of paternity, the substitution of children, and the destruction of the foetus.[17]

Like other categories licensed by the Bishops, such as surgeons, schoolmasters, curates and parish clerks, midwives had to produce local character witnesses, usually the parson and churchwardens of the parish, to testify to the rectitude of their 'lives and conversations'.[18] They also had to bring to the hearing six 'honest matrons' whom they had delivered during their period of instruction and who were willing to testify to their skill. The reliability of this testimony is, of course, difficult to assess. The 'matrons' would be picked cases, and although senior midwives were sometimes brought to bear witness to the candidate's competence, these would be her mistress and fellow midwives. There was no requirement of formal examination as under Continental schemes of regulation, an omission which in 1547 drew unfavourable comment from that much-travelled physician, Andrew Boorde, in his *Breviary of Helthe*.[19] Thus while episcopal licensing may have been reasonably efficient as an instrument of social control, it is doubtful if it was ever more than partially effective as a means of guaranteeing the midwife's professional skill.

A midwife practising on her own account, but without a licence, or one who had otherwise offended against the Act, ran the risk of presentment by the churchwardens of her parish at the Bishop's Court, where she might be prohibited from practice, made to do penance, or excommunicated. But the criticisms of Boorde and others make it clear that despite this hazard many midwives remained unlicensed, as did other practitioners in the wider medical field.[20] The fees for the licence must have been a considerable deterrent to poorer women,[21] and since possession of a licence was not required for practice as a 'deputy' to a licensed midwife, women might continue in this capacity for many years without enquiry into their mode of life. Understandably, the efficiency with which the Act was administered varied with the zeal of the Bishop in discharging his duties.[22] In addition it seems that where unlicensed women were performing a useful service among the poor, it was sometimes judged more appropriate to encourage them to take out a licence than to punish them.

Since this system of licensing was mainly concerned with the midwife's social and religious functions, it was not accompanied by any public provision for her instruction. Nor could many have gained any knowledge privately through books, until the invention of printing made these cheaper and more available. Before this time, English versions of the *De Mulierum Passionibus* by Trotula, the eleventh-century Salerno obstetrician and gynaecologist, had been available in manuscript but it was not until 1540 that the first work on midwifery was published in English. This was *The Byrth of Mankynde*, a translation of *Der Swangern Frawen und Hebammen Rosengarten*, first published in German in 1513 by Eucharius Roesslin, City Physician of Wurms. But the *Byrth* was little more than a restatement of opinions culled from the works of the ancients and, unfortunately, a repetition of their errors. It was only in the seventeenth century, with the publication of English translations of the works of Jacques Guillemeau (1612) and William Harvey (1653),[23] and others, that new knowledge became more readily available. Printed books, however, could only help midwives who could read, and who could afford to buy them, and such women were more likely to be found in the towns than in the countryside, where it appears that many were totally illiterate. According to a later edition of the *Byrth*, 'many ryght honourable ladyes, & other Worshypfull Gentlewomen' had made it their duty to take the book with them to labours and read it to the midwife and assembled company.[24]

As was only to be expected, midwives varied in disposition and in competence. Although, according to the *Byrth*, there were many women who were careful, knowledgeable and sympathetic, there were more who were not:

> for as touchynge mydwyfes/as there be many of them ryght expert/ diligent/wyse/circumspecte/and tender aboute suche busynesse: so be there agayne manye mo full undyscreate/unreasonable/chorleshe/farre to seke in suche thynges/the whiche sholde chieflye helpe and socoure the good women in theyr most paynefull labor and thronges. Throughe whose rudenesse & rashnesse onely I doubte not/but that a greate nomber are caste awaye and destroyed (the more petye).[25]

About midwives' personal circumstances before the seventeenth century not much is known. It is clear that some followed their mothers into the work, some took it up to supplement their husbands' earnings, while others entered it out of sheer necessity. The famous French midwife, Louise Bourgeois (1563–1636), who became midwife to the Queen of France, was about twenty-five when adversity led her to turn to midwifery to support her family; but if contemporary comment is any guide, many were well advanced in years when they first began to practise.[26]

Most probably, the majority had no formal preparation for the work. In his *Observations on Midwifery* Percivall Willughby (1596–1685) said that many, especially in the country, were illiterate women of the 'meanest' sort who, 'not knowing how, otherwise, to live', had taken it up 'for the getting of a shilling, or two'.[27] These women, as the author of *A Companion for Midwives* (1699) put it, practised merely 'upon the privilege of their Age'[28] and most probably, like Dickens' Sairey Gamp three hundred years later, they combined midwifery with sick nursing and laying out the dead, or indeed, any work they could come by to earn their bread. The better class of midwife, however, would spend a period of years working as 'deputy' to an experienced woman before hanging out the sign of the cradle. Sometimes her instructor would be her own mother;[29] if not, her training might necessitate a considerable outlay, like the five pounds paid by the widow Mary Griffen (licensed in 1696) for three years' instruction from Mrs. Anne Slap, 'Ancient Sworn midwife of Deale'.[30] Midwives such as these were to be found in cities or towns, where there were enough families sufficiently affluent to pay the sort of fees which would make an investment in a long training worthwhile. As might be expected, 'professed' London midwives enjoyed the highest status, and had undergone the longest training, in many cases as much as seven years.[31]

Though probably most 'professed' midwives came from the skilled artisan class,[32] there were also 'gentlewomen' among their ranks, some of whom, as their publications show, were capable of a high standard of English. These were women from the middle ranks of society, related to men of the class of apothecaries, surgeons, and schoolmasters. In exceptional cases they may have been connected with families of higher social rank. Examples were the daughter of Percivall Willughby, 'Gentleman', a younger son of the Willughby family of Wollaton Hall near Nottingham, and his kinswoman, Mrs. Willughby, a London midwife 'of much practice, and of good repute with women'. In general, however, the letters, diaries, and memoirs left behind by more substantial members of society contain no reference to any friend or relative who was a midwife.

As with medical practice today, the greatest distinction and profit was to be obtained in London, in attendance on the wealthy merchant class and the resident aristocracy, or, the greatest prize, on Royalty itself. Occasionally a midwife would be chosen to travel abroad to attend English princesses who had made foreign marriages.[33] In rural areas, the wife of the lord or squire would engage a leading midwife from the nearby town who would arrive well before the birth, stay for several days afterwards, and be recompensed accordingly. The poor (that is, the majority of the population) would generally not be able to obtain the services of the more successful midwife. In towns a 'professed' midwife starting out in independent practice would begin by attending poor women, but in the country the latter would have to rely on the local midwife, often accessible only by a long journey over bad roads, or on the friendly help of neighbours.[34]

The fees a midwife received would vary with the wealth of her clients, and with her reputation, which she had to build up over time, working her way up from practice among the poorer classes. Attendance on Royalty was especially lucrative, and might bring lasting reward. In 1469 Margaret Cobb, midwife to the Queen of Edward IV, was granted a pension of £10 a year for life, as was Alice Massy for attending Elizabeth of York in 1503.[35] When Madame Peronne, the French midwife, attended Queen Henrietta Maria in 1630, a hundred pounds was allowed for her diet and entertainment, and a further £300 for her actual remuneration.[36]

Clearly women of this eminence might in time become quite well off. One such was Mrs. Hester Shaw, a prominent London midwife in the mid-seventeenth century. Mrs. Shaw attended the aristocracy, mixed socially with the wealthy citizenry, and was a woman of property. In 1650 she had the misfortune to lose her house and effects in a fire, the result of an explosion of gunpowder in a neighbour's house. As a deposition before the Lord Mayor proved, shortly before the fire she had received over £950 in repayment of a mortgage, and the value which she put on her estate, the product, as she said, of 'above forty years' toilsome gleaning in the way of my labourious Calling', was over £3,000.[37]

Gifts from friends of the family were also an important item in the midwife's remuneration. In a well-to-do household, she would receive substantial tips from the attendant 'gossips', and, as shown in the *Midwives' Just Petition* (a humorous pamphlet written against the continuance of the Civil War) she would be a respected guest at the christening. There, she would not only 'feast high',[38] but benefit also from the generosity of the guests as she went the rounds of the assembled company, the baby in her arms. In 1532 Henry VIII gave £3.6.8d. to the 'norice (the 'monthly' nurse) and the mydwif of Sir Nicholas harvy cheilde', and on a similar occasion in 1530, £3. Entries made a hundred years later in the Household Books of the Howards of Naworth Castle show several gifts of 20s. to Mrs. Fairfax, 'my young lady's midwife'. These sums would, of course, vary with the wealth of the giver and the rank of the recipients. In 1661, when the diarist Pepys, a top Admiralty official, was godfather at a christening, he gave the midwife 10s., but a provincial contemporary of his, the Reverend Giles Moore, records giving 'to the mydwyfe in the drinking bowl 1s'. As shown, gifts would also be made to the 'monthly' nurse who in a substantial family would be engaged to perform the more menial tasks during the birth, and to nurse the mother and infant for the following month. Her standing was much lower than that of the midwife, and Pepys tipped her only 5s.[39]

By this period, however, important new developments had taken place which were to have far-reaching consequences for the future of the midwife. The spirit of enquiry which the Renaissance had brought to other branches of medicine was now being directed to the processes of childbirth, as part of the new scientific study of anatomy. Outstanding among the pioneers in this field was Ambroise Paré (1510–90), surgeon to the King of France. Paré is particularly remembered for his re-introduction of podalic version, a method (known to the ancients) of turning the child in certain cases of malpresentation and delivering it by the feet. Paré's work made possible a greater understanding of the mechanism of labour and the consequent advance in operative obstetrics.[40]

This progress, however, had not come about through the work of midwives. The prestige of the new advances belonged to men, and it was this prestige which was further to encourage their entry into

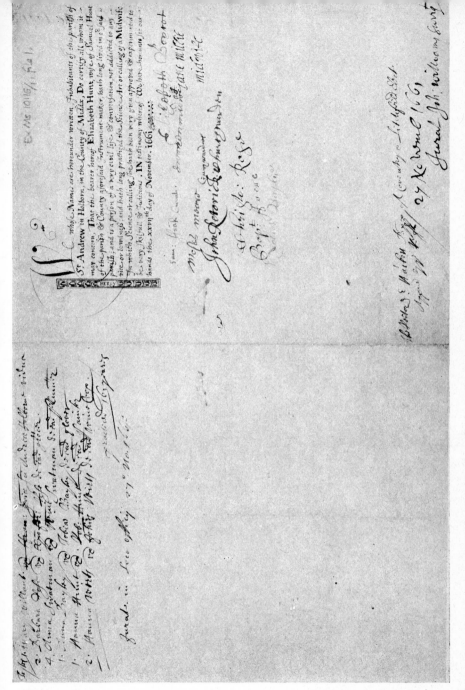

Plate 1

Testimonial relating to the application of Elizabeth Hunt to the Bishop's Court in the Diocese of London in 1661 for a licence to practise as a midwife on her own account. The testimonial is signed by the parish's two churchwardens, the curate, and by two senior midwives who came to testify to the candidate's skill and experience. The names of 'six honest matrons' whom she had delivered and whose testimony was required in support of her application are listed on the left. The signature of John Williams, Surrogate, who acted for the Bishop in granting the licence and administering the oath, appears in the bottom right hand corner.

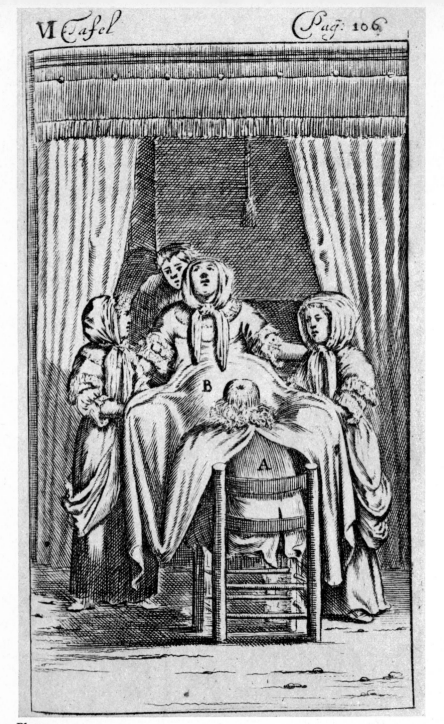

Plate 2

This wood-cut from an eighteenth century Dutch work on midwifery shows
the man-midwife attending a delivery. In the interests of decency he has
the end of the bed-sheet pinned around his neck.

From S. Janson, *Korte en Bondige verhandeling, van de
voortteelingen't Kinderbaren, Amsterdam, 1711, facing page 106.*

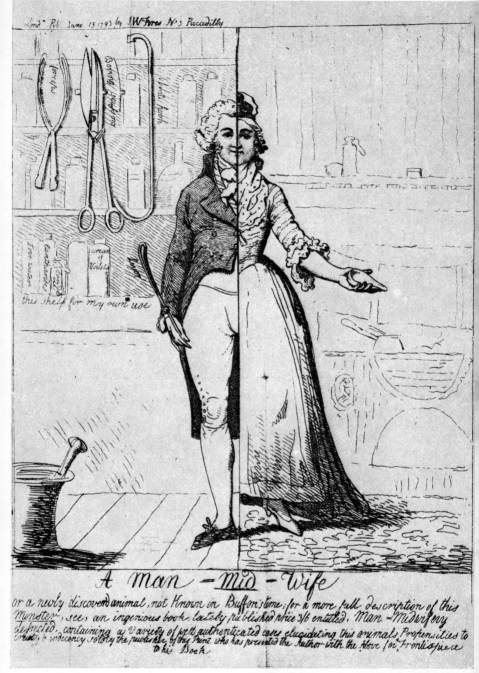

Lond.n Pub. June 15 1793 by SW Fores No 3 Piccadilly

this shelf for my own use

A Man – Mid – Wife

or a newly discover'd animal, not known in Buffon's time; for a more full description of this
Monster; see, an ingenious book lately published price 3/6 entitled Man – Midwifery
dissected, containing a variety of well authenticated cases elucidating this animals Propensities to
cruelty & indecency sold by the publisher of this Print who has presented the Author with the Above for Frontispiece
to his Book

Plate 3

Behind the man-midwife are shown his instruments and bottles
containing the potions which, it was alleged, he used to stimulate
sexual desire in his patients.

From S. W. Fores, *Man-Midwifery Dissected*, London, 1793.

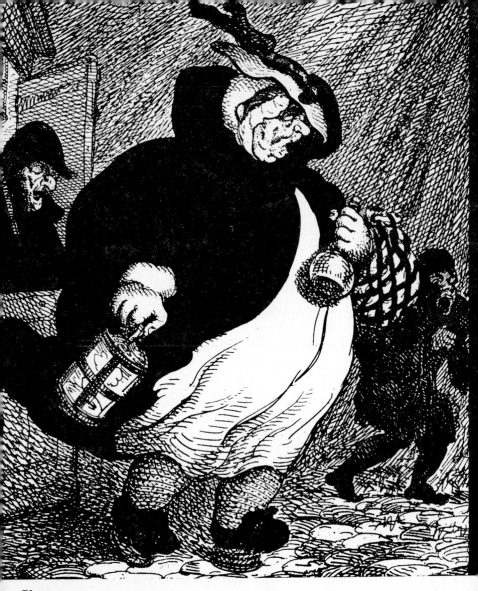

Plate 4
This caricature by Rowlandson (dated 1811) shows a midwife going to a
labour early in the morning, equipped with a lantern and spirit
bottle.

the field of operative midwifery, a development which, as we have seen, had begun in France, but was gradually to become general throughout Europe. In England the existence of this new order of practitioners had been recognized by the early 1600s with the addition of the word 'Man-Midwife' to the English language.[41]

Men-midwives were called mainly to difficult cases, or engaged to be present in readiness for any emergency. However, many women had strong objections to male attendance even in these circumstances, and were, it was said, prepared to die rather than admit a man to the lying-in room.[42] For this reason various strata-gems—not too difficult in the half darkness in which the chamber was customarily kept—might be resorted to. In her 'Instructions to My Daughter' (1617) Louise Bourgeois urged that it should be so arranged that the woman should neither see the man nor know he was there.[43] The man-midwife Percivall Willughby describes such an occasion in 1658. Called in by his daughter, the midwife in the case, he crept into the room on all fours in order to escape detection by the patient, the wife of a Puritan gentleman.[44] Moreover, out of deference to the woman's modesty, the man-midwife commonly worked blind, with his hands under a sheet,[45] a practice which sometimes led to serious error.[46]

Despite recent advances in obstetric knowledge, there was still no public provision in England to help midwives improve their professional competence. Many, as Willughby testified, were dangerously ignorant of anatomy, believing, for example, that the child could be 'stuck' to the mother's back. Often midwives sought to 'help' the birth by forcibly stretching the reproductive parts, sometimes tying the reluctant woman to the obstetric chair, and in more obstinate cases, by tossing her in a blanket, rolling or rocking her, or by other violent measures. It is not surprising that such violence often left the woman with permanent and humiliating dis-abilities, while the ignorance of many midwives in the management of abnormal labour could result in the death of both mother and child.

But mistaken ideas were not the sole prerogative of the midwife. In an age when even scientific and enquiring men like William Harvey thought that the foetus itself, rather than the spontaneous contractions of the womb, provided the motive power for the birth, the belief that the child might need active help in fighting its way into the world must have appeared as an obvious and logical deduction. Harvey condemned the practice of stretching the labia vulvae in the hope of facilitating the birth,[47] and Percivall Willughby, a friend and disciple of Harvey's, describes how when he first took up the work he himself had thought this necessary, but from his knowledge of a number of births which had taken place successfully without any attendant at all, he had since concluded that it was actually harmful.[48] At the same time, for the attendant to dilate the mouth of the womb with the fingers was regarded by some male authorities as a necessary or useful part of routine practice.[49]

Not all the men attracted to midwifery were in the same class as those whose writings have come down to us. Some were the inexperienced young surgeons described by Willughby in his *Observations*; others (even more contemptible in his eyes) were ill-prepared apothecaries. Such men, Willughby complained, 'leaving the beating of their mortars, turn Doctors, as also taking it upon them to bee men-midwives', and yet, despite their fatal ignorance, they escaped the branding-iron and the hangman's noose.[50] There was thus no guarantee that any man setting up as a man-midwife, whether medically qualified or not, really understood his business, any more than there was for the women in this work. Without doubt male practice at its worst was as bad as that of the most ignorant midwife.

Notwithstanding the undoubted evidence on the incompetence of midwives and the rashness of apothecaries and surgeons, there is no way of knowing to what extent their negligence or malpractice was reflected in the maternal death-rate, or, as yet, of estimating what this rate was. John Graunt, who in 1662 made a study of the London Bills of Mortality, and who was well aware of their shortcomings as a basis from which to draw conclusions, nevertheless felt secure in estimating that in London not above three in two hundred 'died in Childbed' (i.e. up to a month after the birth). This figure, though frightening to modern eyes, Graunt evidently found encouraging. Those dying from the 'hardness' of their labour, as opposed to other causes, he considered might number less than one in two hundred.[51] Graunt also agreed with several of his contemporaries that country women living in poor and primitive conditions did best in childbirth.[52] If this were true, it was probably, as Harvey suggests, because poor women often escaped the 'officious' attentions which many midwives thought it their duty to give, and in consequence Nature was allowed unimpeded to take her course.[53]

At this distance in time we cannot know what was the incidence of abnormality in childbirth, though it is possible that rachitic malformation of the maternal pelvis played an important part. It is clear also that if the tugging and stretching to which so many women were subjected did not leave them with permanent injuries, it might well have caused abrasions and lacerations likely to admit the septic infection of the deadly 'childbed' or 'puerperal' fever. There were, it should be remembered, no rubber gloves, and the need for asepsis and antisepsis was totally unrecognized. At the same time all such interference would be undergone without the benefit of analgesics or anaesthetics, and must have resulted in much unnecessary suffering. It was not for nothing that the subsequent ceremony for the 'churching' of women included allusion to the 'pains of Hell' and the 'snares of death'. Such phrases must have seemed no more than a literal description of what she had gone through to many a woman who knelt before the priest with the 'accustomed thank-offerings' for her safe deliverance in the 'great danger of Child-birth'.[54]

Although on the Continent municipal regulation of midwives was by now common, licensing in England remained in the hands of the Church. In 1616, however, proposals were put forward for the establishment of a system of secular regulation for the midwives of London. In that year a group of London midwives petitioned the King to grant a Charter for their incorporation into a 'Society' better to control the standards of midwife practice. 'Through the want of skill in manny w[ch] take uppon them to be midwives', they declared, 'manny women labouringe with child and their children do perish'. It was thus 'very needfull', that

> the skill of the most skillfullest in that profession should be bettered and none allowed but such as are meete which cannot be performed unless the said midwives be incorporated into a Societye.[55]

Following the pattern of the Physicians' and Surgeons' corporations, this body would have provided lectures for its members and supervised and regulated their practice. A midwives' corporation, however, would have been a complete innovation, since, probably in consequence of the family ties which still hamper the organization of women workers today, in no country do midwives seem to have had their own guild. Nor does it appear that the proposals would have given the midwives themselves actual control over their own Society. Though ostensibly the plan had originated with them, it was in fact the brain-child of the man-midwife Dr. Peter Chamberlen, surgeon to the Queen. Chamberlen belonged to the remarkable Huguenot family which invented the midwifery forceps—an invention which, from motives of self-interest, they were to keep to themselves for the next hundred years. This same self-interest evidently played a large part in Chamberlen's proposals for the midwives' corporation, which were carefully designed to give him the powerful position of 'Governor' with the lucrative monopoly of licensing and instructing the members and attending their calls in difficult cases.

The scheme for the Society was referred by the King's Privy Council to the College of Physicians for comment. But the College, while it admitted the need for improving the practice of midwives, 'whoe for the most parte are very ygnorant', held it 'neither necessary nor convenient' that they should be elevated to the dignity of a self-governing corporation, 'a thinge not exampled in any common-wealth'. In their view, the matter could be adequately dealt with by requiring all midwives seeking a Bishop's licence to be first examined and approved by the College. The College could also provide any necessary instruction, including, once or twice a year, 'dissections and anatomyes to the use of their whole companye'.

With the Physicians against the proposed incorporation, Chamberlen's scheme was bound to fail. The College's own suggestion for the instruction and examination of midwives was not taken up, however, and in 1634 Chamberlen's nephew Peter, aged thirty-three, revived the proposal for a midwives' Society. Again midwives petitioned the King, and again their request was opposed by the Physicians. This time, however, opposition came also from among midwives themselves. Over sixty other London midwives, under the leadership of Mrs. Shaw and Mrs. Whipp, had organized resistance to the Chamberlen bid to assume control over them and their livelihoods.

Chamberlen, the objectors complained, was not to be trusted with any project for midwife regulation, since as a man-midwife he had a pecuniary interest in being called to cases which midwives could not manage, and thus more to gain from keeping them ignorant and incompetent than from encouraging them to improve their practice. For this reason 'unsufficient' midwives had become Chamberlen's 'deare daughters', who

> oftentimes by their bungling and untoward usage of their women, and ofttimes through ignorance do send for him, when itt is none of his worke, and so to the damage of the partie both in body and purse do highly increase his profitts.

Further, the consent of those midwives supporting his proposals had not been freely given. Chamberlen had bribed some by entertaining them with 'Venison, wine and other delicates', at the same time threatening that if they did not comply with his wishes he would no longer answer their emergency calls. Moreover, it was mere presumption for Chamberlen to propose to instruct midwives, since he lacked the necessary experience of natural labours, he himself delivering none 'without the use of instruments by extraordinary violence in desperate occasions'. As for his suggestion that he should teach them anatomy, this was quite redundant, as they themselves had text-books on the subject written in English, 'which would direct them better (most of them being able to read) then [sic] his learned Lectures'.

The dissident midwives briefed counsel to represent them at the official enquiry into the petition, held before the Archbishop of Canterbury. There they had the satisfaction of seeing Chamberlen not only fail in his efforts to gain control over midwives, but himself have to seek a licence for the practice of midwifery from the ecclesiastical authorities whose efficiency he had called into question. But although opposed to Chamberlen's proposals, Mrs. Shaw and her colleagues were themselves not satisfied that episcopal licensing was functioning as effectively as it should. Complaining that many ignorant women were practising without a licence, they appealed to the Court to 'timely direct a remedy and carefully proceed in the admittance of midwives in the future'.[56]

Notwithstanding this request, things evidently continued much as before, and in 1647, during the suspension of episcopal licensing under the Commonwealth, the resilient Chamberlen again returned to his criticisms of the episcopal system. On the testimony of 'two or three Gossips', he protested, any woman, however ignorant or cruel, who took the oath and paid her fee, would be licensed to practise. 'But of Instruction or Order amongst the Midwives', he complained, 'not one word.' It was high time that the regulation of English midwives should be removed from the Church and made the duty of some civil authority.[57]

Although the midwives who had opposed Chamberlen's scheme had expressed their concern about the number of uninstructed women in the work, it was not until 1671 that the first text-book written by an English midwife was published. This was the *Midwives Book*, by Mrs. Jane Sharp of London, 'Practitioner in the Art of Midwifery above thirty years',[58] and evidently a well-read and much travelled woman. Addressing herself to her 'Sisters, the Midwives of England', Mrs. Sharp gave her reasons for writing the book, the product of her study of foreign authors and her own experience:

> I have often sat down sad in the consideration of the many Miseries women endure in the Hands of unskilful Midwives, many professing the Art (without any skill in anatomy which is the Principal part effectually necessary for a Midwife) meerly for Lucres sake.[59]

But although her book contains much good sense, it is shot through with the superstitions of the age, and is not in the same class as the valuable *Observations* written fifty years before by Louise Bourgeois,[60] midwife to the Queen of France. Still less does it compare with the outstanding contribution made to the subject a few years later in the work of the celebrated Justina Siegemundin, midwife to the Court of Prussia, whose method for dealing with arm presentations still bears her name.[61]

But it was not only midwives who were still in the grip of superstition. Some of Mrs. Sharp's quaint beliefs were shared by educated men like Mauriceau, Sermon, and even the hard-headed Willughby, whose sovereign remedy for a flooding was a draught made of hog's dung and ashes of toad, helped out by poultices and pessaries of similar composition.[62] When the man-midwife Jules Clément attended the Dauphine in 1682, he bled her at regular intervals during the thirty hours of the labour. Afterwards he had recourse to an ancient remedy which was thought to promote recovery after a hard delivery. The Dauphine was wrapped in a newly-flayed sheep-skin—which, to the horror of her ladies, had been taken off the live animal in the actual lying-in chamber. Then, since to allow the mother to sleep immediately after a difficult birth was considered dangerous, she was forcibly kept awake for several hours. Finally, although this was in the middle of an August heat-wave, her room was sealed up, and she stayed in bed without even the light of a candle for nine days.[63]

By this time male practitioners were also writing for midwives. In his *Ladies Companion, or, The English Midwife*, 1671, Dr. William Sermon lays down what qualities a midwife should possess:

> As concerning their Persons, they must be neither too young, nor too old, but of an indifferent age between both; well composed, not being subject to diseases, nor deformed in any part of their body; comely and neat in their Apparell, their hands small, and fingers long, not thick, but clean, their nails pared very close; they ought to be very chearfull, pleasant, and of a good discourse, strong, not idle, but accustomed to exercise, that they may be the more able (if need requires) to watch, &c.
>
> Touching their deportment: they must be mild, gentle, courteous, sober, chast, and patient, not quarrelsom, nor chollerick; neither must they be covetous, nor report any thing whatsoever they hear or see in secret, in the person or house of whom they deliver; for, as one saith, it is not fit to commit her into the hands of rash and drunken women, that is in travel of her first Child.
>
> As concerning their minds; they must be wise, and discreet; able to flatter, and speak many fair words, to no other end, but only to deceive the apprehensive women, which is a commendable deceipt, and allowed, when it is done for the good of the person in distress.[64]

Other men-midwives concurred in this general opinion, as they did in their definition of a 'good' midwife as one who sent for a man in difficult labours, and who was not so 'lofty and conceited' that she used instruments herself.[65] While this may have been good advice to midwives who were unable to manage such cases themselves, and who lived in places where an experienced man was available, it also had the merit for the male practitioner of advocating a course best calculated to serve his own pecuniary interests.

Old Mrs. Sharp herself had been shrewd enough to see which way the wind was blowing. Although at this period men attended only difficult or abnormal births, the position of the midwife was already threatened by their advent on the scene. Since many midwives lacked both theoretical and practical knowledge, Mrs. Sharp feared that men might come to be preferred to women on account of their undoubted educational advantages:

> Some perhaps may think, that then it is not proper for women to be of this profession, because they cannot attain so rarely to the knowledge of things as men may, who are bred up in Universities, Schools of learning, or serve their Apprentiships for that end and purpose, where Anatomy Lectures being frequently read, the situation of the parts both of men and women and other things of great consequence are often made plain to them.

However, this objection could 'easily' be answered, she thought. Although for the foregoing reasons men might 'in some things' attain to greater perfection, with long and diligent practice women could also gain 'farther knowledge', which they could then communicate to their own sex.

It was indicative of the way things were going that Mrs. Sharp felt the need to defend women's prior claim to midwifery. Midwives were recorded in the Bible, she pointed out, 'to the perpetual honour of the female Sex'; men-midwives, however, were not so much as mentioned. Although conceding the honour due 'to able Physicians and Chyrurgions, when occasion is', Mrs. Sharp could not forbear poking fun at the pretensions of those gentlemen for their use of Latin and Greek terms, reminding them that it was not 'hard words' that performed the work, 'as if none understood the Art, that cannot understand Greek'. Among all 'barbarous' peoples, where there were no 'Men of Learning', women were adequate for the work; 'and even in our own Nation' . . . the 'poor Country people', assisted only by women, 'are as fruitful, and as safe and well delivered, if not much more fruitful, and better commonly in Childbed than the greatest Ladies of the Land'.[66]

But as Mrs. Sharp admitted, it was much more difficult for women to acquire the anatomical knowledge necessary for good practice. The better-trained midwives certainly studied anatomy and saw dissections, but even they did not enjoy the same opportunities as men. Men were free to travel abroad to the great continental seats of learning, where these studies could be pursued further; such travel would not have been possible for unattended women, and, except in Italy, the universities were closed to them.

Moreover, the general educational opportunities open to women were greatly inferior to those enjoyed by men. Grammar schools and universities were open only to boys, and charity schools for girls aimed at fitting them for the more humble occupations. Finally, the private boarding schools springing up in response to the desire of tradesmen to purchase gentility for their daughters gave only a very superficial education, concentrating largely on needlework, fine cooking and 'accomplishments'. It is not surprising that, as Willughby testifies, few midwives were proficient in foreign languages,[67] or in Latin, in which many medical works were still written and from which so many medical terms were derived. Mrs. Sharp could afford the expense of having texts translated,[68] but even the best midwives must have been at a disadvantage both educationally and socially compared with men of the calibre of Willughby and Harvey, and, however competent, were unlikely to enjoy equal prestige.

But midwives suffered a further handicap. Even at the close of the seventeenth century European tradition still required that they should be married women of mature age, who had borne children. It was because of her childlessness that Justina Siegemundin came near to being rejected for the post of Midwife to the City of Leignitz.[69] For this reason women taking up midwifery would generally be older than their male counterparts, and would be well past their learning 'peak'. They were also likely to be hampered by domestic ties, another factor militating against that complete commitment which is an essential pre-condition of scientific discovery and advance in any field. Furthermore, in a climate of opinion which actively discouraged literary efforts by women,[70] it had to be an exceptional midwife who would find the determination, as Mrs. Sharp had done, to write for her fellow practitioners.

On the Continent, Government was already active in the provision of instruction for midwives and in many German cities there were formal arrangements under which physicians or midwives were specially appointed for this work.[71] In France, too, there had been an important advance in the matter of midwife instruction. In 1631, the great public hospital in Paris, the Hôtel-Dieu, had begun to take a small number of pupils, an opportunity, however, not offered to men, except to a few native or foreign surgeons enjoying Royal patronage. In keeping with tradition, 'apprentisses' had to be married women or widows, and to profess the Catholic faith. Their training lasted three months, during which time they received instruction in anatomy and watched dissections.[72] In England, however, the only improvement was the more general availability of text-books in the vernacular for those without a classical education.

Nor could England boast any provision for lying-in women such as existed at the Hôtel-Dieu. However, in 1688 a proposal for the foundation of lying-in wards in London was put forward by a midwife, Elizabeth Cellier. A few years earlier Mrs. Cellier had gained notoriety for the part she had played with friends of the Duke of York (now James II) in the Catholic 'Meal Tub Plot'. In consequence she had stood trial for treason, but had defended herself so ably that she had been acquitted. Subsequently, however, she had over-reached herself. Her pamphlet '*Malice Defeat'd*', was adjudged a seditious libel, and she was sentenced to appear twice in the stocks and to pay a fine of £1,000.

Mrs. Cellier now turned to the improvement of midwives. With the Restoration had come the return of episcopal licensing, which, according to Mrs. Cellier, was no more a guarantee of skill than it had ever been.[73] Her own remedy, like that of the Chamberlens, was to incorporate all the skilful midwives of London into a Midwives' College, which would provide for the instruction and supervision of members and furnish a forum for the discussion of professional matters. Besides this, the College itself was to finance another new venture, a Royal Foundling Hospital, with twelve associated lying-in houses for the accommodation of pauper women sent there by the Overseers of the Poor.[74]

Mrs. Cellier's scheme had many impractical features, and, like Chamberlen's earlier one, was no doubt intended to secure advancement for its proposer. Yet the foundation of a self-governing Midwives' College could have done for the status of midwives what their own corporations were to do for surgeons and apothecaries. However, the proposal evidently met with similar objections among physicians as the Chamberlens' earlier scheme, namely, that there was no precedent for a Midwives' College, and that Mrs. Cellier's plan was merely an amusing pretension on the part of a midwife. Mrs. Cellier defended her scheme with her usual vigour. Associations of women physicians, she insisted, had existed in antiquity, dedicated to the female deities, and midwives were certainly 'antienter' than doctors.[75]

But even if King James had looked with favour on the project, as Mrs. Cellier claimed, it is more than likely that the College of Physicians would have been as opposed to a self-governing midwives' corporation as it had been in 1616, and would have been successful in blocking it. Under continental systems of regulation, midwives were clearly subordinate to physicians and surgeons, and in Paris the 'Maîtresses sages-femmes' had recently lost their long-standing right to participate in the examination of midwife candidates.[76] In Ireland, the power to license midwives, shortly to be given to the King's and Queen's College of Physicians under their Charter of 1692, made clear the midwife's inferior position.[77] As it turned out, however, King James was forced to go into exile the following year, and episcopal licensing remained the only form of midwife regulation throughout England. By contrast, in Scotland the Edinburgh Town Council was in 1694 to follow the continental example with the institution of a system of municipal licensing[78] which was to continue for a large part of the following century.

All this time more and more men were entering midwifery. This was particularly so in France, where male practice was much more firmly established than elsewhere. As early as 1617 Louise Bourgeois had protested about the 'coquettes' who engaged men-midwives even for normal labour,[79] and in 1680 the fashion for their routine employment had received further encouragement from Louis XIV's engagement of Jules Clement for attendance on the Dauphine. From then on the 'bonnes bourgeoises' had followed the great Court ladies in seeking male attendance.[80]

But in England, as in the rest of Europe, men were still employed only in emergencies, or, in wealthy households, to wait in readiness for such eventualities.[81] Thus despite the clouds which Mrs. Sharp had detected on the horizon, at the close of the seventeenth century midwifery in England remained almost completely a female occupation, and one which, moreoever, the educated gentlewoman fallen on hard times might take up with the prospect of earning an honourable livelihood.

CHAPTER TWO

The Decline of the Midwife

The eighteenth century was a period of great change. Agrarian improvements, the move to industrialization and urbanization, the increase in population, and the growth of prosperity all had far-reaching effects on people's lives, and especially on those of women. In the middle of the century women were still largely engaged in productive work in their own homes, often acting as their husbands' partners in craft-work, business or agriculture. Over the next hundred years, however, the change to large-scale farming and the decline in domestic industries made this less and less possible. At the same time, the womenfolk of newly prosperous tradesmen and farmers increasingly left the counter and the dairy for a life of leisure in the parlour—a poor qualification for earning a living should the future leave them unprovided for. Finally, the continuing professionalization of other occupations, as for example, medicine, worked gradually but inevitably towards the exclusion of women.[1]

Even in the traditionally female occupation of midwifery, women were losing ground. From the 1720s onwards, more and more men were coming into the field. Moreover, they were no longer only called in to attend abnormal labours, but were beginning to be engaged for routine cases. In consequence they were now in direct competition with the midwife. Thus work which since time immemorial had been the preserve of women, and in particular the resort of women with families to maintain, was gradually being lost to men.

There were several reasons for this change. As already noted by Jane Sharp, 'Men of Learning' who took up this work had higher status than midwives, irrespective of their skill. The distinction of the great men-midwives of the eighteenth century—men like Richard Manningham, Fielding Ould, William Smellie and William Hunter —was to reflect credit on every male practitioner, whether deserved or not. However, it was probably the introduction of the midwifery forceps, a development which occurred about 1720,[2] which precipitated this rapid acceleration in what was already an existing trend. The forceps enabled its user to deliver live infants in cases where previously either child or mother must have been lost, and also to shorten tedious labour. It thus gave the doctor or surgeon an additional advantage over the midwife (to whom custom did not allow the use of instruments as an accepted part of her practice) and so further enhanced the position of men.[3]

As in France, fashion played an important role in this process. Writing in 1724 in his *Female Physician*, John Maubray observes that the 'Politer Part of the World' had already begun to put themselves in the hands of men. Soon the 'middling classes' were following suit, and by the 1760s the practice was spreading to the tradesman and artisan class.[4] In this, as in many other occupations, men generally received higher remuneration than women; it was therefore important to the aspiring tradesman to show his neighbours that he could afford the higher-priced article.[5] Moreover, the growing prosperity of the times meant that increasing numbers were able to do so.

While these foregoing factors all favoured the male practitioner, another development worked directly to depress the midwife's standing in the community. Although episcopal licensing had been designed primarily as a means of social control, it had also served to confer status on the women who were licensed. But now, as the power of the Church waned, this system was breaking down. In London and surrounding areas it had ceased to operate by the 1720s, and although persisting longer in the provinces, in some places into the early 1800s,[6] it seems generally to have disappeared by the last quarter of the century. Even where licences were still granted, it does not appear that any prosecution of unlicensed persons took place, and, as with the midwife in *Tristram Shandy*, licences appear to have been sought purely for the official cachet they conferred,[7] rather than as an essential preliminary to practice.

In Scotland and Ireland more attention was given to midwife regulation than in England. In 1726 Edinburgh had strengthened its law relating to midwife regulation and in 1740 the Glasgow Faculty of Physicians and Surgeons instituted a system of examination and licensing for midwives in the city and surrounding counties, which, as in Edinburgh, appears to have operated until the end of the century. Steps were also being taken for a similar system of midwife regulation in the New World. In 1716 the New York Common Council had passed an ordinance requiring midwives to take out licences, and to swear a version of the traditional midwives' oath.[8]

Scotland was also to be first with provision for midwife training.

In 1726 Edinburgh Town Council had appointed a Professor of Midwifery, Joseph Gibson, the first such appointment in the British Isles. It is probable, however, that Gibson also took male pupils. From the standpoint of the young surgeon or apothecary, the attraction of midwifery was the entrée it gave to medical practice proper. Once admitted to the lying-in room, the man-midwife might well become medical attendant to the whole family,[9] and many surgeon-apothecaries had in fact become 'general practitioners', though the term itself was not yet in use. By the middle of the century 'several hundred' men-midwives (though this may be an exaggeration) were said to be practising in London and its environs, and there was also a practitioner 'of standing' in every large town.[10]

As was to be expected, midwives viewed this trend with alarm. Clearly, the only way to arrest the progress of men, some of whom were anxious to drive women from the work altogether,[11] was to raise the general level of female practice. It was out of this concern for her 'Sister Professors in the Art of Midwifery' that in 1737 Mrs. Sarah Stone, a Taunton midwife who had later moved to London, published her *Complete Practice of Midwifery*. This was the product of her thirty-five years' experience in the work, and Mrs. Stone hoped that it would enable women even 'of the lowest capacity' to deliver their patients successfully without 'in every little seeming difficulty' calling in a man. Unless women showed themselves capable of dealing with difficult cases, she warned, the public would send for a man in the first place, as was already the fashion with the ladies of Bristol. Thus, merely for the lack of good 'Women-Midwives', practice would pass entirely to men, and 'the Modesty of our Sex will be in great danger of being lost'.[12]

Like Jane Sharp before her, Mrs. Stone stressed the importance to the midwife of a thorough grasp of the relevant anatomical knowledge, reassuring her readers that it was 'not improper' for 'all in the Profession' to read anatomy or see dissections, as she had done. But thorough practical experience was also necessary; for 'had I inspected into them [dissections] all my Life, and had not been instructed by my Mother, and Deputy to her full six years, it would have signified but little'. Every midwife should therefore spend at least three years 'with some ingenious Woman' to learn her work; 'for if seven years must be served to learn a Trade, I think three years as little as possible, to be instructed in an Art where Life depends'.[13]

But it was not only midwives who objected to the growth of male practice. Opposition existed in the ranks of medicine itself, as shown by John Douglas' *Short Account of the State of Midwifery in London, Westminster, &c.* published in 1736. Douglas was a well-known

London surgeon, and brother to James Douglas, the eminent man-midwife. Though Douglas himself saw a role for men in abnormal midwifery, he considered that such work belonged properly to the surgeon, and that physicians and apothecaries who practised it were trespassing beyond their province. Moreover, in order to strengthen their hold on the work, male practitioners were insisting that mid-wives should call in a man 'in every trifling little difficulty', reducing them to the condition of 'mere nurses'. Yet male assistance was not always available, even in London; and in the country, where mid-wives were more ignorant, it was often out of the question. Besides this, for reasons of modesty many women would not agree to send for a man, nor would their husbands allow it. More would refuse because they could not pay his fee, which, indeed, was often de-manded beforehand. Why, then, asked Douglas, did not men, instead of forever blaming and rebuking midwives, do their best to instruct them as thoroughly as possible?[14]

Douglas' comments on the attitudes of male practitioners to the subject of midwives' instruction were not without justification. Though Edmund Chapman and other male writers for midwives expected that a midwife should be capable of certain manual operations, most were adamant that she should not use instruments. Moreover, in Thomas Dawkes' *The Midwife Rightly Instructed* (1736), a work written in the form of question and answer between surgeon and midwife, the surgeon refuses to tell the midwife how to deal with a haemorrhage. Even her objection that in country areas there may be no apothecary to whom she may send for medicines fails to move him. Warning her not to aspire *beyond the capacities of a woman*, he replies, 'I never designed, Lucina, to make you a Doctress, but to tell you how to practise as a Midwife.'[15]

This refusal to give women full instruction on the ground of their alleged incapacity to deal with difficult cases, was scornfully dis-missed by Douglas as mere 'artful and groundless insinuation'. All ages had produced their learned women, as well as their illiterate, thick-headed physicians; it was not native deficiency, therefore, but the want of adequate instruction which disabled English women in the performance of this office. If proof of female ability were wanted, it could be found in the career of Madame du Tertre, a past Head Midwife of the Hôtel-Dieu, whose text-book for midwives demon-strated her status in the field.[16] English midwives, Douglas con-tended, could certainly reach the same standards if they had the opportunities available to Frenchwomen. Recognizing the important part played by the Hôtel-Dieu in the training of French midwives, he demanded the establishment of lying-in hospitals in all the principal cities of England.[17]

Douglas was not the only one to deplore the lack of such provision in England. Three years later, in 1739, a beginning was made by a leading London man-midwife, Sir Richard Manningham, with the institution of a 'Charitable Infirmary' for the relief of poor married women in two wards of St. James' Infirmary, Westminster. Hitherto, Manningham explained in the advertisement of his Charity, 'due Knowledge' of the practice of midwifery could not easily be obtained without going abroad, which for most pupils, especially women, was out of the question, with the result that they were not as fully qualified for their business as they should have been. However, it was as much Manningham's object to provide instruction for men as for women, and accordingly both sexes were admitted as pupils at the Hospital. Indeed, Manningham hoped that as the necessary knowledge had now 'come home to them', more young practitioners would study midwifery.[18]

It was also Manningham's hope that before too long Parliament would recognize its duty to establish a *National* Hospital which would serve *all* lying-in women, single and married alike. Until then, however, his 'little temporary one' would relieve married women only. But when in the next decade permanent lying-in hospitals were established (Manningham's institution does not appear to have lasted long)[19] they were the product not of Government action, but of the remarkable upsurge in organized private benevolence which was already making so much charitable provision for other categories of need.

The first of these permanent institutions was the Lying-in Hospital in Dublin (later the 'Rotunda Hospital'), founded in 1745. This was followed by the establishment of lying-in wards in the Middlesex Hospital in 1747, and the foundation of the British and City of London Lying-in Hospitals in 1749 and 1750. Next, in 1752, came the hospital in Jermyn Street (the 'General Lying-in Hospital'— later, the 'Queen's Hospital', and, still later, 'Queen Charlotte's'), and in 1765, the Westminster New Lying-in Hospital (in the nineteenth century known as the 'General Lying-in Hospital'). In Edinburgh, lying-in wards were opened in the Royal Infirmary in 1756. Dependent on public subscription, these institutions were of necessity small affairs, and it is likely that in their early years all the London hospitals together made less provision for lying-in cases than did the Hôtel-Dieu in Paris, where nearly fifteen hundred women were delivered each year.[20]

Like the voluntary general hospitals and other charities springing up in major towns, lying-in hospitals resulted in part from the initiative of medical men seeking a ready source of clinical material for their own and their pupils' study. But they were also an achievement of the active humanitarianism of the increasing numbers of affluent middle-class philanthropists, of whom the Thorntons, the Hoares and the Whitbreads were such outstanding examples. Such men saw the provision of hospitals as a duty, to be undertaken not only out of compassion for the 'distressed objects' of their charity, but also in the interests of their particular class and of the nation at large. The poor, potential subscribers were reminded, were the 'Riches of the Rich', and the 'Instruments of the Ease and Happiness of the Community'. They were also—and this was an important consideration in view of current fears that the population was falling —the source from which the fleets and armies for the defence of the country and its growing foreign acquisitions were supplied.[21]

The benefits of the first London lying-in hospitals were available, free of charge, to poor married women 'of good character', though the Westminster Hospital and the General Lying-in Hospital admitted single women pregnant with their first child. These hospitals were designed to serve the wives of soldiers, sailors, 'poor industrious Mechanics' and 'distressed Housekeepers' (householders). To qualify, applicants had to be fortunate enough and respectable enough to obtain from a hospital subscriber one of the limited number of letters of recommendation available. They also had to come to the hospital cleanly clad and free of vermin and contagious disease.

Women seeking free attendance, but unable through poverty or other reasons to satisfy these conditions, had to apply to the Overseers of the Poor. Such women (if they were not victims of the strenuous efforts so often made by the Overseers to whisk out of the parish any 'great-bellied' woman without a settlement there)[22] would be cared for in the workhouse, if one had been built, or possibly in an inn, or in their own homes. The parish would pay for the attendance of the midwife (in some parishes a man-midwife might be called to difficult cases)[23] and often for nursing during the lying-in.

Like other voluntary charities, lying-in hospitals were run by Boards of Governors elected from among the subscribers. The 'Gentlemen of the Faculty' gave their services free, reaping the reward of public recognition in their private practice. The day-to-day running of the hospital, and responsibility for normal deliveries lay with the Matron—always a widow. For her exacting labours she received an annual salary of £25 to £30, plus board and lodging, —equivalent to that of a housekeeper or lady's maid in a fairly well-to-do household. She was clearly subordinate to the Medical Officers, in whose hands was the overall responsibility for the patients, and whom she had to call in to abnormal labours.[24] In addition, the Medical Officers were also members of the Weekly

Board which appointed and dismissed paid staff. The Matron's position thus contrasted unfavourably with that of the Head Midwife at the Hôtel-Dieu, who was independent of the medical staff and who called in the surgeon only when she considered instruments were necessary.[25]

Despite this, the lying-in hospitals were to play an important part in the future of the midwife, since in most of them instruction was available for women, though at a price. At the British Lying-in Hospital which, like the City of London, took no male students, the 'Gentlemen of the Faculty' gave theoretical instruction 'in all that is necessary for Women to know' for a fee of twenty guineas a head. Pupils had to pay a further ten shillings a week for board and lodging, 'exclusive of Tea, Sugar and Washing', and there may also have been fees to the Matron, who was responsible for practical training. All in all, including the cost of travel to London (the British Lying-in Hospital prided itself on serving the whole country), this must have amounted to more than £30 for a minimum stay of four months. Although this compared favourably with premiums paid for apprenticeships for young girls in millinery and dress-making,[26] it was still a considerable sum for a married woman or a widow with a family to find, unless, as was the case with Mrs. Wood, the midwife in *Tristram Shandy*, her training was financed by a local benefactor.[27] It was probably for this reason that the Hospital appears never to have taken its full complement of twelve pupils a year, averaging at most between three and four.

Following general custom, the British Lying-in Hospital required its pupils to be married women or widows; they also had to be at least twenty-five years of age, and of good character. In general they came from the skilled tradesman class, being the wives or widows of shoemakers, tallow-chandlers, carpenters, maltsters, masons, butchers, and the like. Occasionally, there was the wife or widow of a farmer, an upper servant in a gentleman's household, or a minor government official. A few were married to apothecaries or surgeons,[28] and once in a while there was a clergyman's widow, or the wife of a 'Gentleman', or of a junior army officer, presumably in reduced circumstances.

But as far as the actual provision of skilled assistance to lying-in women was concerned, a greater contribution was made by the out-door charities which sprang up in London and provincial towns in the second half of the century. Many of the free dispensaries offering general medical services also attended midwifery patients, while other charities, like the London Lying-in Charity (later the Royal Maternity Charity) were created solely for this purpose.[29] Some lying-in hospitals also opened out-door departments. The general pattern was for patients to be routinely attended by mid-wives working under the general supervision of the institution's man-midwife, whom they had to call in to difficult cases.[30] Out-door charities were not responsible for boarding, lodging, or nursing their patients; in consequence their costs per patient were lower, and the number of women attended by their midwives greatly exceeded the number delivered in hospital.[31] Moreover, since outbreaks of child-birth fever were a frequent occurrence in hospitals, out-door patients were without doubt far safer.[32]

Some of the larger out-door charities also trained midwives. These were women from a similar social background to the pupils of the lying-in hospitals, but the instruction they received was free. In return for their training, the midwives worked for the charity for an agreed period at specially low fees of 1s. 6d. or 2s. od. the case, compared with the half-a-crown or five shillings paid by the Over-seers of the Poor for Poor Law work. At the same time, they were free to take up private practice, and the charities took pride in the service which they were providing to the community by training women for work generally among the poor and 'middling' classes.[33] In some country parishes the squire or parson might finance a midwife's training, as did Parson Yorick in *Tristram Shandy*, or even pay her a small salary for attending the poor.[34]

By this time male practice appears to have been increasing more rapidly than ever,[35] arousing bitter hostility from those who saw this new development, along with many others, as a change for the worse. Opposition came not only from the midwives whose livelihood was in danger, but also from leading medical figures and from members of the general public. The more vocal of these opponents expressed their views in books, pamphlets and letters to the press. Though their more extreme opinions were probably shared only by a small minority, the repeated appearance and sale of similar publications during the next hundred years was to indicate a continuing opposition to man-midwifery.

To these adversaries of male practice its growing popularity had nothing to do with superior skill on the part of men. In his '*Man-Midwifery Analysed*', the journalist Philip Thicknesse attributed it solely to a slavish desire to follow Fashion. Once this French practice had been adopted by a few aristocratic ladies with negligent hus-bands, complained Thicknesse, the 'middling classes', who always felt bound to 'ape the quality', had copied them in this as in every-thing else.[36] However, the Queen herself still set an example to the nation in being attended by a midwife.[37]

But there was another factor. Men-midwives, it was said, anxious to establish their own importance in the eyes of the public, took every opportunity of helping Fashion do its work. To this end they exaggerated the dangers of childbirth and frightened women into believing that extraordinary measures, and therefore male attendance, were more generally necessary than they actually were. At the same time they made the most of every occasion to denigrate the understanding and competence of midwives, and to blame them, however unjustly, for anything that went wrong.

Finally, the male practitioner consolidated his position by making an ally of the monthly nurse. If a midwife were not employed, the nurse would not have to share the customary gifts from the attendant 'gossips'; moreover, the man-midwife, anxious to win her good-will, might even tip her as well. By this means, writes Thicknesse, 'he convinces Mrs. Nurse *almost* to the bottom of her heart, that a female midwife is as dangerous about the person of a lying-in woman, as a rattlesnake about a man's leg: she sounds the Doctor's trumpet far and near; and all her kind mistresses, and indulgent masters are sure to have the warmest recommendation of Dr. Blowbladder's art of touching'.[38]

The man-midwifery controversy received light-hearted treatment at the hands of the novelist Sterne. In *Tristram Shandy*, with its comical figure of the 'scientific operator', Dr. Slop, Sterne caricatures the well-known practitioner, Dr. Burton of York. As Sterne observes, 'Human nature is the same in all professions', and Dr. Slop, like many members of emergent professional groups, is anxious about his status. Except on the occasion when he cuts his thumb and forgets to stand on his dignity, he rejects the homely, intelligible title of 'man-midwife', insisting on the newly fashionable French 'accoucheur'. Annoyed that the old midwife has been put in charge at Tristram's birth, and that he himself has been engaged only to wait in case instruments should be needed, the doctor cannot forbear asserting his superiority over her when the occasion offers. When, to his satisfaction, the midwife does ask for his assistance, he refuses to go upstairs to her, but demands that she come down to him. At the same time he takes the opportunity—unjustifiably, in view of her long years of successful practice—to belittle her in front of the Shandy family. Finally he applies his favourite instrument, the 'new-invented forceps', and in so doing crushes the bridge of Tristram's nose.

Other comment was less restrained. Some of the publications condemning male practice were clearly intended by their journalist authors to titillate the public appetite for salacious stories and so ensure commercial success. For this reason they appealed to the age-old male fear that any relaxation in customs affecting women was likely to weaken wifely fidelity, from which it was only a short step to the collapse of society and the constitution of the State.[39]

One of the chief proponents of this view was Francis Foster, the puritanical author of *Thoughts for the Times but Chiefly on the Profligacy of Our Women* (1779). Here Foster rehearsed his anxieties about the decline in female virtue. The increasing number of divorces, he complained (then about three a year[40]) showed how far moral deterioration had progressed. Boarding-school education, French novels, and French dances like the cotillion and the allemande, all had their corrupting effect on women. But of all the pernicious influences at work in society, man-midwifery—which gave the enemy direct access to the very citadel of female virtue—was by far the worst.[41]

The argument was an old one, deriving from a fundamental male anxiety concerning supposed feminine weakness and inconstancy, and was a favourite among extreme opponents of the male practitioner. A woman handled by the man-midwife became 'polluted', and, in consequence, more likely to admit other men to similar familiarities.[42] Indeed, argued Thicknesse, if men-midwives were to resist all the temptations to which they were inevitably exposed, they had to be *more*, or *less* than ordinary men. Yet it was well known that under the sanction of the physician's 'great wig' and 'grave face', they took every opportunity to seduce their patients, travelling from one conquest to another 'like the Emperor of Morocco, or the Bashaw of Tangier, going to his seraglio'.[43]

The possibilities for amorous dalliance between the man-midwife and his patient had not escaped the ballad-writers, and in *The Man-Midwife Unmasqu'd* (1739) 'Doctor D. . . .' is sued by a patient for rape. But although the Doctor had certainly taken advantage of the situation, he did not suffer in consequence. The jury, justly entertaining doubts about the plaintiff's own innocence in the matter,

> . . . return'd the Bill 'Ignoramus'
> And the Doctor has now got a Name that is famous.

How far men-midwives did succumb to their patients' charms is, of course, impossible to say, and Thicknesse's claim that the records of 'every court in the kingdom' would confirm his allegations[44] about the 'Touching Gentry' was no doubt exaggerated. One case of this sort did attract a great deal of notice, however, and was to provide the opponents of male practice with useful ammunition for a long time to come. This was an action for 'criminal conversation' brought in 1741 by a wealthy London merchant, George Biker, against a Dr. Morley. The doctor had attended Biker's young and handsome wife in a miscarriage; later he had taken advantage of his subsequent acquaintance with the family to seduce her. The wife (possibly as a result of mental distress following the discovery of her adultery) died shortly afterwards in a madhouse, and the husband was awarded damages of £1,000. But like the doctor in the ballad, Dr. Morley's practice does not seem to have been adversely affected by the publicity. In 1754 he was spoken of as a 'Physician of great Eminence in his Profession', and was substantial enough to have a further £1,000 damages awarded against him on account of his fatal negligence in a midwifery case.[45]

But if the attendance of men-midwives was open to such grave objections, so, protested their opponents, was the practice of allowing male students to learn their profession in the wards of lying-in hospitals. Even if the only patients they attended had forfeited their claim to virtue (the General and Westminster Lying-in Hospitals admitted single women), it was wrong to subject such wretched, frightened, harassed women to the indignity of being constantly available to the 'inspection and palpation of a set of youths'. Nor was it right to expose these 'poor young pupils' to such shockingly indecent temptations to wantonness.[46]

Another continuing theme in the attack on men was their 'abuse' of instruments. Here, without doubt, the man-midwife's opponents were on stronger ground. The man-midwife Willughby had complained of this rashness over eighty years before and a strongly worded denunciation had appeared in 1724 in Dr. John Maubray's *Female Physician*:

> However I know, some Chirurgeon-Practitioners are too much acquainted with the Use of *INSTRUMENTS*, to lay them aside; no, they do not (it may be) think themselves in their *Duty*, or proper *Office*, if they have not their cruel Accoutrements in Hand. And what is most unaccountable and unbecoming a Christian is that, when they have perhaps wounded the *MOTHER*, kill'd the *INFANT*, and with violent *Torture* and inexpressible *Pain*, drawn it out by Piece-meal, they think no Reward sufficient for such an extraordinary Piece of mangled Work.[47]

Similar admonitions figured in the writings of later practitioners, and the celebrated William Hunter is said to have shown his students his forceps, rusty from disuse, with the warning that 'where they may save one, they murder twenty'.[48]

This point had been strongly urged by Sarah Stone in her *Complete Practice of Midwifery* in 1737. Of recent years, she alleged, more mothers and children had died at the hands of raw recruits just out of their apprenticeship to the barber-surgeon than through the worst ignorance and stupidity of midwives. Yet by adopting a 'finished assurance', and claiming that their knowledge exceeded any woman's, these young 'Gentlemen-Professors' so secured their position that '. . . if Mother, or Child, or both, die, as it often happens, then they die *Secundum Artem*; for a Man was there, and the Woman-Midwife bears all the blame'.[49]

In 1751 the argument was forcibly restated in *A Petition of the Unborn Babes*, a pamphlet by Dr. Frank Nicholls, Physician to George II, and an eminent member of the College of Physicians. In the *Petition* the 'Babes' accuse men-midwives of 'wickedly' building their fortunes by preying on the ignorance of women and frightening them into engaging a male practitioner. Yet by their own misuse of instruments they were themselves often guilty of the death of both mother and child. Accordingly, the 'Babes' appealed to the Censors of the Royal College of Physicians for protection against these abuses.[50]

According to William Hunter, Nicholls' attack on men-midwives was motivated by jealousy of their success, 'because we get money, our antagonists none'.[51] Be that as it may, Nicholls himself is reputed to have profited from the exercise. It is said that as Mrs. Kennon, midwife to Queen Caroline, lay on her death bed, she gave Nicholls a bank-note for £500 for his services to the midwives' cause. These services did not stop with the *Petition*, however, and the following year Nicholls proposed to the College of Physicians that the College itself should offer instruction for midwives. This should take the form of an annual course of free lectures, for women only, 'to render them as fully qualified in point of Knowledge to assist in Labour and the Disorders incident to Breeding Women as they are fitted for it by the Caution, Patience, Tenderness, and Decency natural to their sex'.[52] He himself offered the sum of £1,000 towards the cost, again said to have been donated by Mrs. Kennon. But the College showed no interest in the proposal and it was allowed to die.

Nine years later, another midwife, Elizabeth Nihell, published her contribution to the controversy—a 400-page polemic against male practice under the title *A Treatise on the Art of Midwifery*. Mrs. Nihell, who lived with her surgeon-apothecary husband in the Haymarket, was unusual in that she had obtained the privilege, rare for a foreigner, of training at the Hôtel-Dieu. There the midwives worked without male supervision or intervention, and from her observation of their successful practice she had concluded that instruments were seldom, if ever, necessary. On one occasion, she recalled, the Head Midwife, Madame Pour, had delivered a two-headed monster without recourse to instruments and with the help of no-one but a pupil midwife.[53]

Mrs. Nihell's views on instruments were shared by Thicknesse and by other opponents of male practice. The man-midwife, they argued, was for 'dispatch'. He used instruments unnecessarily to hasten the birth and save his own time, as well as to impress the family with his dexterity and justify charging a higher fee.[54] Consequently more infants were lost than formerly, and if the mother did not die of the injuries she might sustain or of resulting childbed fever, she was frequently left with fearful and lasting disabilities.[55] Worse still, complained Mrs. Nihell, the male practitioner, adding insult to injury, was so adept at concealing his errors with 'a cloud of hard words and scientific jargon', that the injured patient herself was convinced that she could not thank him enough for the mischief he had done.[56]

These onslaughts on man-midwifery did not pass without rebuttal from male practitioners, who could be as guilty of employing exaggeration and cheap sensationalism as were their opponents. Midwives were ignorant beldames, alleged one, who not only crammed their patients with cordials, but in order to hasten the birth drove them up and downstairs or subjected them to violent shakings, all the while ridiculing them and making fun of their distress. These 'doting dram-drinking matrons' wrote another, had lost every womanly quality but weakness of understanding and the wretched prejudices of the old wife. Many women suffering from incontinence, or from a fallen womb, had cause to regret their reliance on 'these worst of women'.[57]

What degree of truth there was in these allegations and counter-allegations is at this distance in time impossible to determine. Educated midwives certainly possessed the anatomical knowledge essential to good practice. In general, the standard of the best London midwives is likely to have been higher than elsewhere, and some of them, as critical medical testimony indicates, were extremely well qualified.[58] But the bulk of midwives were limited to lowly paid attendance on the poor. Such practice did not attract women with a good educational background who could afford to invest money in learning a profession. It followed therefore that the majority must be drawn from the lower classes in society. These women would have had little opportunity to acquire real knowledge of the processes of childbirth and many of them would have been full of the ignorance which so often led to rash and fatal interference.

Better-educated midwives prided themselves on maintaining high standards both in their professional and private lives. Advising mid-wives on their general conduct in her *Domestic Midwife* (1795), Margaret Stephen, a London midwife of long experience, warned them never to accept cordials, 'though oft invited to do so'. Nor would she allow these to be given to the patient[59]—a practice deplored by another educated midwife, Martha Mears, in her *Pupil of Nature* (1797) as still very prevalent, particularly among the lower classes.[60] Mrs. Stephen also dealt with the charge that midwives were always women of drunken habits and low moral character:

> Those who have found it in their interest to bring midwives into disrepute, have charged them with intemperance, and even obscenity. How the being a midwife should make women possess such vices, is to me a mystery. I know no way of life in which a woman can be engaged, that is more calculated to fix sentiments of piety and morality upon the mind, nor have I ever been acquainted with any midwife who did not possess them.[61]

Yet the figure of the drinking midwife (like that of the nagging mother-in-law today) had long been part of traditional folklore. In Shakespeare's *Twelfth Night*, written two hundred years before, Maria rejoices with her conspirators that her plot against Malvolio is working 'like aqua vitae with a midwife'. Since most midwives were older working-class women, they could be expected to share the drinking habits usual in women of their age and station. At this time, too, drinking played a much larger part in the everyday life of all ranks of society than it does today, old customs requiring that many little occasions should be marked by drinking or treating. When a woman went into labour, her 'gossips' were sent for post-haste—day or night—and at the consequent gathering there was often more merriment than at a feast. In these circumstances it is not surprising that patients were often encouraged to partake liberally, especially as alcohol was widely believed by public and doctors alike to have great medicinal and strengthening properties.[62]

But the midwife had a long-standing and unsavoury reputation of another kind—that of a manager of sexual intrigues—'truest friend to lechers', as the seventeenth-century poet Rochester put it.[63] Some of their number, like 'the Amphibious Necessary, between Bawd and Midwife', in Ned Ward's *Rise and Fall of Madam Coming-Sir*, were procuresses, or worse.[64] Many, like the 'Mother Midnight' of Defoe's *Moll Flanders*, ran private lying-in homes (as, indeed, did some men-midwives also) where 'ladies of pleasure', or others anxious to keep their pregnancy hidden, might be aborted, or await the birth of their child in secret. Here the proprietress' arrangements with the Overseers of the Poor would protect them from persecution or punishment by the parish officers—always anxious to prevent within their boundaries the birth of a child likely to become chargeable to the rates. The unfortunate child would then be disposed of, sometimes, as in *Madam Coming-Sir*, murdered on the premises, or, perhaps, put out to nurse. There were always women who for a down payment would take a child on the understanding that no questions would be asked about its welfare, and with whom its expectation of life was likely to be short. Then, if she had no protector, the young mother might be set to work as a prostitute for the proprietress for as long as she was useful.

As far as relative safety between male and female practice was concerned, there was insufficient information on which to base accurate comparisons. However, enough evidence existed to suggest to one thoughtful medical enquirer that common assumptions about the superior safety of male practice might be open to question. In his *Treatise on the Management of Pregnant and Lying-in Women*, Dr. Charles White, himself a well-known man-midwife, pointed out that although the poor were often half-starved and diseased, and served only by ignorant midwives, their maternal death-rate might still be less than that of patients delivered in lying-in hospitals, or of the more affluent class attended by men.[65]

Whatever the rights and wrongs of the controversy, the growth in male practice continued unabated, increasingly taking the better paid work from midwives. To make matters worse, the old tradition that men should be paid at a higher rate for the same work applied in midwifery as in other spheres. In 1760, making an early protest against unequal pay, Elizabeth Nihell had condemned this devaluation of the midwife's work. No matter how expert or assiduous a midwife might be in her care of the mother before and after the lying-in, she declared, or how attentive to the welfare of the child, 'so seldom regarded by the men-midwives', many people felt they could never pay her too little, '*for no other reason on earth, but because she is not a man*'.[66]

Men-midwives, she complained, fanned these prejudices, arguing that midwifery was a 'manual operation' and therefore better suited to men; furthermore, that it actually degraded the art to allow women to practise it. Yet the truth was the very opposite of this. Not only did women have more compassion for their sex's sufferings, but their hands, being softer and more supple, were less likely to cause discomfort to the patient undergoing internal examinations than the boisterous 'grabbling and rummaging' of the 'delicate fist of a great horse-godmother of a he-midwife'. Moreover, women had patience to wait on Nature, whereas men frequently used instruments to save their time, often damaging the mother and killing the child. Yet although it was only because of this 'glorious privilege' of using instruments that men had attained to their 'usurped office', they now had the blasphemous effrontery to maintain that work which God himself had given to women was fitter for men.[67]

The jealousy of male competitors, alleged Mrs. Nihell, was chiefly directed against the more successful midwives who represented the greatest threat to their advancement. There were many French surgeons who had been glad to take lessons from leading Parisian midwives, yet some of them, far from acknowledging their debt with respect and gratitude, had not scrupled to belittle female capacity and intellect. Even so, it had to be admitted that too few midwives were sufficiently mistresses of their profession. Some, like many men-midwives, were of a very low level of competence, but with the difference that they were incapable of doing as much actual mischief. All midwives, she stressed, should be thoroughly grounded in the anatomy relevant to their work and be able successfully to undergo the most rigorous examination in this subject. At the same time, the only way to exclude 'ignorant practitioners of either sex' was to subject both men and women practising midwifery to a system of governmental regulation such as obtained in Holland, with the prohibition of practice by all unqualified persons.

Mrs. Nihell warned her readers that the future of the midwife was in real danger. Already 'false prejudices' against midwives were discouraging suitable women from taking up the work and replacing those good female practitioners who had 'gone off the stage'.[68] Thus the time might well come when, despite all the obvious objections to employing men, the public would be forced to this because there were no competent midwives to be had. However, it was not only the occupation of midwife which was at stake, but the whole field of women's work. There had never been enough employment for women, Mrs. Nihell pointed out, but now, as the result of the decrees of Fashion, occupations which had formerly belonged to them were increasingly invaded by men. But where would men stop? After the injustice of driving midwives out of their livelihood, what professions would they leave to women? If this trend continued, she protested, 'it will at last be discovered that men can spin, raise paste, cut out caps, pickle, and preserve, better than we do'.[69] It was fortunate for women that there was no prospect of the occupation of dry-nurse becoming as lucrative as that of the man-midwife. Otherwise, Mrs. Nihell concluded,

> I should not dispair of seeing a great he-fellow florishing a pap-spoon as well as a forceps, or of the public being enlightened by learned tracts and disputations, stuffed full of Greek and Latin technical terms, to prove, that water-gruel or scotch-porridge was a much more healthy aliment for new-born infants than the milk of the female breast, and that it was safer for a man to dandle a baby than for an insignificant woman.[70]

Mrs. Nihell's assessment of the market for women's labour was correct. In consequence of increasing industrialization, which in many trades separated the workshop from the home, much gainful work was lost to the woman tied to her house and family. At the same time men were also invading other traditionally female employments. The fitting and making of women's stays had already gone to men, and ladies' hairdressing, which in the past had given many London women 'genteel bread', had now been taken over almost entirely by the fashionable, and more expensive, 'French Barber', or by men who, by speaking broken English, passed for such.[71] Moreover, as prosperity increased it was becoming less and less respectable for women to work outside the home, or even in the family business. More and more tradesmen sent their daughters to boarding schools to learn French and 'accomplishments', and, as Defoe had commented with disapproval in his *Compleat Tradesman*, kept their wives and daughters in the parlour rather than the shop. Such a climate did not encourage women of good educational background to take up work like midwifery.

Yet in the 1770s some London midwives were apparently making over £1,000 a year and keeping 'elegant' carriages.[72] However, as the *Gentleman's Magazine* pointed out, most of those recommended by the author of one of the pro-midwife pamphlets lived in mean courts and lanes.[73] This may, as Mrs. Nihell suggested, have been in part accounted for by the public's expectation that even highly skilled midwives should receive less than men, but was probably also due to their failure to attract a better-paying clientele. Indeed, the advice given by Margaret Stephen to her pupils on fees to be charged might, if followed, have earned them the gratitude of the poor, but would certainly not have advanced their success in the eyes of the world. 'Be always ready', urged Mrs. Stephen,

> to the calls of distress, and do not stand out because you do not know how you are to be paid. Never distress the distressed, nor turn your back upon a patient because she is become poor, and raise not your demands because you are come into great practice. If circumstances admit, people will be ready to put a proper value upon your time; and where you think they do not, you should be delicate in telling them of it, for some may think they have given as much as you should expect, though you are of a very different opinion. Avarice is a very bad qualification, or rather a bad vice, in those who have the health and life of their fellow creatures under their care.[74]

As the century wore on, so the decline of the midwife continued— a cumulative process accelerated by the interested propaganda of a section of the medical profession, and in particular, of younger men anxious to capture the midwifery which gave the entrée to general practice. Mrs. Stephen relates how she herself had suffered from such calumny. In a case where the patient's friends, impatient of the delays of a tedious but normal delivery, had demanded that a man be called in, it was not the experienced practitioner whom she recommended who was sent for, but a young, untried, and *cheaper* man, whose clumsy efforts with the unnecessary forceps killed the child. Despite her tact in helping him conceal his error from the company, 'this perfect twig of the obstetric profession' had put the blame on her, and in consequence became the valued medical attendant of this 'little Plebeian family'.[75]

Midwives should therefore take care, warned Mrs. Stephen, not to put their patients, or their own reputation, at the mercy of young and inexperienced men;

> . . . for had this affair happened in the earlier part of my practice, it might have hurt me very essentially, as *then*, like most of the *profession*, I was employed in the lower walks of life: and as the ignorant are always very credulous, the charge of having been the occasion of a child's death, would in all probability have tript my heels.[76]

Leah Cousins, the successful and honoured village midwife described by George Crabbe in *The Parish Register* (1807), was not so lucky. Crabbe, who had himself trained as a surgeon, describes how the town-bred wife of a young farmer,

> A gay vain bride, who would example give,
> To that poor village where she deigned to live

engaged, in preference to the midwife, a newcomer to the village, 'young Dr. Glibb'. Despite the fact that he lost the child, the wealthier part of the village were so impressed by his claim that it was only his skill that had saved the mother, that they left Leah and went over to him.[77]

The young doctor did his best to help on this process, sneering at Leah as 'Nature's Slave', who trusted only to luck, and in emergencies to prayer, while he, with his 'skill' and 'courage', took pleasure in bending Nature to his will. In reply Leah pointed to her long record of success:

> That I have luck must friend and foe confess,
> And what's good judgement but a lucky guess?
> He boasts, but what he can do: will you run
> From me, your friend! who, all he boasts, have done?
> By proud and learned words his powers are known;
> By healthy boys and handsome girls my own:
> Wives! fathers! children! by my help you live;
> Has this pale Doctor more than life to give?
> No stunted cripple hops the village round;
> Your hands are active and your heads are sound;
> My lads are all your fields and flocks require;
> My lasses all those sturdy lads admire.
> Can this proud leech, with all his boasted skill,
> Amend the soul or body, wit or will?

But it was no use; her 'truth was vain', and gradually she declined and died, embittered and poor, deserted by those whom she had served so well.[78]

Most defenders of the midwife had always been aware of the need for adequate instruction for women, especially in anatomy, and midwives who put themselves under men teachers were warned to beware lest they were cheated. Male practitioners, it was alleged, anxious to suppress female practice among the rich, taught midwives less thoroughly than their male pupils, in order to foster their dependence on men, and so discredit them in the eyes of wealthy patients. In short, they trained midwives for their own service, not for that of the public.[79]

This warning was repeated by Margaret Stephen in her *Domestic Midwife*. She herself demanded high standards from her pupils, expecting them to consult the works of leading authorities like Smellie, Baudelocque, and others. Male teachers, she complained, took larger fees from women (the usual fee was ten guineas) yet taught them less, and then proclaimed to the world that women were ignorant and not to be trusted. For this reason she promised to continue with her own lectures to midwives 'until the men who teach that profession render them unnecessary by giving their female pupils as extensive instruction as they give the males'.[80]

The theoretical grounding which she gave her pupils was evidently very thorough. Her lectures included

the anatomy of the pelvis, &c, and of the foetal skull, on preparations which I keep by me, with every thing else relative to practice in nature, at labours; also turning, and the use of the forceps, and other obstetric instruments, on a machine which I believe few teachers can equal; together with the cases and proper seasons which justify such expedients; and I make them write whatever of my lectures may prove useful to them, in their future practice, for which they are as well qualified as men.[81]

But although she taught the use of forceps, she advised midwives always to send for a man when these were necessary, explaining that where the outcome was unfortunate, 'people are more reconciled to the event, because there is no appeal from what a doctor does, being granted he did all that could be done on the occasion'.[82]

Like many others who during the century had expressed their concern about the condition of midwives, Mrs. Stephen urged the need for a public examination which would distinguish the qualified woman from the unqualified.[83] Most advocates of regulation, however, wished to go further than this and prohibit all unqualified practice, both male and female. Demands for such regulation had come alike from midwives, medical men, and members of the lay public. Significantly, medical advocates of regulation proposed that midwives should be placed under medical control through the London corporations of Physicians or Surgeons. Midwives and their supporters, on the other hand, with equal significance, proposed regulation by lay governmental authorities.

As far as the training of midwives was concerned, this was still left to voluntary charity or private endeavour, and in this field, as in others, charitable organizations multiplied during the second half of the century. Notable among these was the Manchester and Salford Charity, later St. Mary's Hospital. Founded in 1790 by Dr. Charles White, it aimed at creating a 'School or Nursery of Young Midwives' for providing the town and surrounding counties with women of knowledge and experience. In contrast to the London lying-in hospitals, the Charity provided free instruction to its own out-patient midwives and other pupils. In 1796 its example was followed by the Liverpool Ladies' Lying-in Charity, which appears to have been run on similar lines, though it was unusual among charities of this size in that its managing committee consisted entirely of women. England, however, compared unfavourably with Scotland, where in Edinburgh alone over a thousand midwives had been trained between 1780 and 1818,[84] or probably more than four times the number produced in the four London lying-in hospitals combined.[85]

Active steps were also being taken in Ireland for the improvement of midwife practice. In 1765 the Irish Parliament had empowered Grand Juries (the County authorities) to provide funds for the establishment of County Hospitals. Twenty years later, as part of its general policy of rate support for health care (Ireland had no Poor Law) the Juries were empowered to raise a rate of £30 every five years to send a midwife for training at the Rotunda in Dublin.[86]

Yet despite the increasing emphasis on training midwives in Edinburgh, the regulation of midwife practice in both Edinburgh and Glasgow appears to have broken down by the end of the century. On the Continent, however, regulation and instruction was still very much the concern of governmental authority. Many German towns had special 'Hebammenmeister', or teachers of midwives, and also midwives' schools.[87] In France, where there was growing apprehension that the population was falling, the central government had been attempting to improve the practice of provincial midwives, most of whom, as in England, were said to be very ignorant. In 1770 the King's Physician, Joseph Raulin, was commissioned by the Government to publish a text-book for their instruction,[88] and the Government also sent the eminent midwife, Madame Ducoudray, on a tour of the provinces to lecture to midwives and to organize the establishment of lying-in hospitals.[89]

After the Revolution, the Government of Republican France was equally anxious to encourage population growth, and in 1803 embarked on determined measures to improve midwife practice in the country at large. Under a comprehensive national system of medical regulation set up that year, midwives were divided into two classes—the 'first class', who might practise anywhere in France, and the 'second class' who were licensed for practice in their local department. At the same time, departmental prefects were required to finance local women as pupils at the Paris 'Maternité' (the successor to the lying-in wards of the Hôtel-Dieu) where training, now to last six months, had been reorganized under Government regulations. No less than eighty women took the first course,[90] or nearly as many as were being trained annually in the lying-in hospitals of the whole of the United Kingdom eighty years later.[91]

French and German midwives thus benefited from government recognition, government regulation, and government-provided and subsidized instruction, all lacking in England. Though the defenders of the English midwife recognized the need for better instruction, they cherished the unrealistic hope that this would be furnished either by midwives themselves, or by voluntary charity.[92] But, as Mrs. Nihell had made clear, educated women would only invest in training for work which promised adequate rewards; once this prospect disappeared, recruitment from this class would fall off and ultimately cease. Nor was the continuance of a body of competent, educated midwives in itself a compelling enough object to attract charitable funds. This was to come only later, when the plight of the unsupported middle-class woman, no longer able to turn for a livelihood to midwifery and other dwindling employments, had become sufficiently acute to arouse public attention. Until that time, the decline of the English midwife would continue without interruption, and male practice would become more general in England than anywhere else in Europe.

CHAPTER THREE

The Ascendancy of Men

During the eighteenth century the man-midwife had advanced from being merely an attendant on the emergencies of childbirth to gaining a hold on the greater part of the best-paid midwifery. Many male practitioners had achieved distinction and respect for their work; and two of their number, Manningham and Ould, had been knighted. At the same time, by taking up midwifery, surgeon-apothecaries were making it *de facto* a part of medicine. Yet in the medical hierarchy where the old divisions of Physic, Surgery and Pharmacy were still officially recognized, the man-midwife as such had no place. This anomalous position made him an easy target for his enemies, who held him up to ridicule as merely a 'mungrel' physician, who had only invaded the province of women because of his inability to succeed in medicine proper. His very name—'Man-Midwife'—was a contradiction in terms as ridiculous as his practice.

Neither the College of Physicians nor the Company of Surgeons were anxious to accept these new practitioners into the fold. Soon after the dissolution of the Barber-Surgeons' Company in 1745, the new Company of Surgeons had passed a bye-law prohibiting members who practised midwifery or pharmacy from election to the Court of Assistants, its governing body, thus effectively limiting control of the Company's policy to the small and fortunate élite who could make a living from surgery alone.[1] The College of Physicians, which since 1783 had honoured a few distinguished men-midwives by conferring on them a 'Licence in Midwifery', in 1800 ceased this practice, and four years later followed the Surgeons' example in passing a restrictive bye-law banning men-midwives from election to its Fellowship.[2]

The real reason for this policy of exclusion was the low regard in which the practice of midwifery was still held by the medical Establishment. This contempt was shared by many of the general public, and even at the end of the century the feeling was still strong. The wife of James Hamilton, Professor of Midwifery in Edinburgh from 1800 to 1839, found her presence at a charity ball objected to on the grounds that the wife of an accoucheur was 'unfit company for respectable ladies and gentlemen'.[3] In 1823 this same prejudice worked to the disadvantage of Sir William Knighton, Keeper of the Privy Purse to George IV, when Lord Liverpool refused to make him a Privy Councillor. A man who had been 'accoucheur to all the ladies in London', Lord Liverpool considered, was not fit for this honour.[4]

The totally unregulated state of midwifery did not help. Though throughout the eighteenth century proposals for the regulation of male *and* female practice had been put forward by both medical men and midwives, nothing had been done. In 1797 an attempt had been made to persuade the Surgeons' Court of Assistants to take a lead on this question when the Company applied for a new Charter. The Court had been requested by a group of the Company's members to abolish the restrictive bye-law, and at the same time to institute a qualification in midwifery.[5] This request was not granted, however, and it was not until 1851 that the Surgeons finally agreed to change their policy on these points.

But if the Court of Assistants was reluctant to set up a qualification in midwifery for men, it was even more determined to have nothing to do with midwives. If the Company were to examine women, it was argued—and at the same time abandon its restrictive bye-law— nothing could stop midwives from becoming eligible for election to the Court of Assistants. In fact, any midwife who could pass such an examination would have been of a much higher class than most women in the occupation. But by conjuring up visions of Lincoln's Inn Fields swarming with the drunken blowzy old hags (like the one caricatured by Rowlandson in Plate 4) its opponents could easily laugh out the whole idea of midwife regulation. The following extracts from verses attributed to Okey Belfour, Clerk to the Company, make the Court's attitude on the subject very clear:

> But when to the Court
> The Clerk made his report,
> And came to this part of the tale,
> All the members astound
> Looked indignantly round,
> And with rage and vexation grew pale.

> Mr. Hawkins spoke first,
> And he look'd fit to burst,
> If the face a man's feelings reveals,
> And he vowed that no power
> Should consort him one hour

With old women in Lincoln's-inn-fields.

. . .

Next to him Mr. Howard,
Neither peevish nor froward,
Who his sentiments never conceals,
Said such nasty old sluts,
With their prominent guts,
Should ne'er rump him in Lincoln's-inn-fields.[6]

In 1808 another approach was made to the College (by the terms of its new Charter the Company had been elevated to this dignity in 1800) and simultaneously to the College of Physicians, to see if either body would set up a qualification in midwifery for both men and women. This time the initiative was taken by a group of London accoucheurs under the leadership of the distinguished Dr. Denman. Again the attempt failed. The Physicians' answer was predictable; they had jurisdiction over persons prescribing medicine, but none over those practising the 'Manual Part of the Profession'.[7] The Surgeons contented themselves with expressing their concern over the problem, while explaining that they had 'no Authority to interfere'.[8]

But it was not only in midwifery that proposals for reform were being put forward. Since the breakdown of episcopal licensing there had been no national system of regulation in any branch of medicine. Now, however, increasing dissatisfaction among those medical practitioners holding formal qualifications led to new proposals for the regulation of the profession. The initiator was Dr. Edward Harrison, a Lincolnshire practitioner, who together with local colleagues had undertaken an enquiry into the extent of unqualified practice in the county. Unqualified practitioners, he discovered, exceeded the formally qualified by as many as nine to one—a proportion which subsequent investigations in other areas were to show was not unusual. Seldom, if at all, was a midwife found who had received any instruction.[9]

It was to remedy this state of affairs that Harrison joined with sympathetic members of the College of Physicians and Surgeons to press for a national scheme for medical regulation, somewhat after the pattern of the new system instituted in Republican France in 1803. The reformers' object was to lay down qualifications for entry to all branches of medicine, and to suppress unqualified practice. Besides embracing chemists and veterinary surgeons, their scheme catered for the examination and licensing by local medical boards of both men *and* women practising midwifery[10]—a plan which might have done much to raise standards among midwives, especially in the countryside. On the other hand, it would have placed them under the control of men who were also their rivals for practice in the same locality. In the event, however, the whole proposal proved too radical for the profession's leaders, and Harrison was forced to acknowledge failure.[11]

In 1812 the matter was taken up yet again. This time the initiative came from a group of apothecaries, who had formed themselves into the 'Association of Apothecaries, Surgeon-Apothecaries, and Practitioners of Midwifery'. Surgeon-apothecaries, that is, men holding both the Licence of the Apothecaries' Society and the Diploma of the College of Surgeons, now constituted the majority of the regular profession.[12] Many of these also practised midwifery. Indeed, according to one correspondent of the *Medical and Physical Journal*, it was 'impossible' to keep up a country practice without it.[13] It was about this time that the new term 'general practitioner' came into use to describe the growing numbers of medical men combining these three functions.[14]

Originally formed to protest against the increased tax on glass bottles, the Association decided to widen its scope and campaign for legislation for the regulation of the profession and the suppression of unqualified practice. Anxious to shed their old association with trade and foster a new image of the apothecary as a member of 'a scientific and liberal profession', the Association was concerned in particular to prevent 'encroachment' on their preserves by the rising class of druggists, many of whom also visited and prescribed for the sick.[15] Their plan, which was similar to Harrison's, and like his, included arrangements for local medical control of midwifery practice, male and female, gained more support, being introduced as a Bill into the Commons in 1813. But again the scheme proved too far-reaching for the three London medical corporations, and because of their opposition, the Bill was withdrawn.[16]

Despite this, a measure of reform did result from the Association's efforts, albeit indirectly. Eventually the Apothecaries' Society itself was persuaded to introduce a more limited measure, dealing solely with the regulation of apothecaries. This passed into law as the Apothecaries Act in 1815. The Act laid down the qualifications to be required of all persons intending to practise as apothecaries, and the penalties for unqualified practice. Moreover—a new departure— it undertook this for the whole of England and Wales. But although the majority of qualified medical men practising midwifery were Licentiates of the Society,[17] the Act did not require them to possess a qualification in this branch—a great disappointment to the Associated Apothecaries, for whom the regulation of midwifery practitioners, both male and female, had been one of the principal objects of their campaign.[18]

As the Apothecaries Bill was going through Parliament, the College of Surgeons, evidently encouraged by the Bill's expected success, speedily introduced their own measure in an attempt to secure parallel privileges relating to the practice of surgery. This new Bill also contained no provision for the regulation of midwifery, and it was only after strong representations from the Associated Apothecaries that the College reluctantly agreed to include a clause requiring that in future all men-midwives should hold its diploma in surgery—no guarantee, however, of their competence in midwifery. The question of providing for the regulation of *midwives* was raised in the Commons Committee which discussed the Bill, but the Members would not entertain the idea.[19]

The Bill made swift progress through the Commons, but because of the lateness of the season proceeded no further and was not revived until three years later in 1818. By then the favourable climate had changed. The Commons showed themselves sceptical about the alleged dangers of unqualified practice, and the Surgeons were accused of having mere monopoly as their aim. Voicing the Free Trade principles which had motivated the recent repeal of the Elizabethan Act providing for regulation of apprenticeship and wages, the House declined to give the Bill a second reading.

The next attempt to obtain the regulation of midwifery came in 1826, from a group of London midwifery lecturers headed by Dr. Augustus Granville who had formed themselves for this purpose into an Obstetrical Society. The Society's object was to secure some recognized system of instruction and regulation by putting pressure on the English medical corporations and, if necessary, on the Government. Midwifery, the Society pointed out, was part of the medical curriculum in the University of Edinburgh and in the principal Universities on the Continent. Yet in England only a small minority of the students destined to practise it had any instruction, theoretical or practical, in the subject.[20] Further, an officially recognized midwifery qualification would serve to distinguish the medical man who had qualified himself for the work from the rest of the profession, and also from the 'self-made' practitioner without any qualification at all. One of these, a Rochdale man prosecuted by the Apothecaries in 1823, had gone straight from working fourteen hours a day in a woollen mill to practise as an apothecary and man-midwife.[21] Another, a 'broken barber's clerk', had recently requested one of the Society's members to give him a paper certifying him as qualified in midwifery.[22] For the protection of the 'subordinate classes', who could not afford the fees of the regularly qualified man, the Society suggested that such 'empirical' practitioners should be subject to licensing by municipal authorities. There was, however, no mention of midwives.[23]

The reformers had some success with the Apothecaries' Society, who agreed to include midwifery in their examinations as soon as they were empowered to do so. The reaction of the Physicians and Surgeons, however, was as negative as before, and it was only after a second request from the Society that the Surgeons agreed to demand certificates of attendance at midwifery lectures from candidates for their diploma. Though the Society sought the help of Sir Robert Peel, the Home Secretary, it had to rest content with these limited concessions. Then, since from the very first its members had stated that they did not wish to set up any body which might lead the public to view them as a class of practitioners separate from the rest of the profession, the Society was disbanded.

The attitude taken by the Colleges of Physicians and Surgeons on the matter had clearly revealed the extent of the prejudice still current in the governing bodies of these institutions against men practising midwifery. Defending the Physicians' ban on the election of accoucheurs to the Fellowship of the College, its President, Sir Henry Halford, explained to Sir Robert Peel that it should not 'create surprize' that midwifery, being a manual operation, was 'deemed foreign to the habits of Gentlemen of enlarged academical education'. In any case, an educated background was not necessary to the successful practice of midwifery, and 'discreet Matrons' and 'plain uneducated men in the Country', often achieved considerable repute without it.[24] Sir Henry was later staunchly to defend this opinion to the Select Committee on Medical Education in 1834.

Similar views were held by Sir Anthony Carlisle, a member of the Council of the College of Surgeons, and later its President. Sir Anthony had argued strenuously against the College's making any concession on midwifery education, but had been defeated. He was not willing to stop there, however, and in May 1827 he wrote a long letter to *The Times* condemning man-midwifery in general and in particular the Obstetrical Society's efforts to 'regularise' their 'dishonourable vocation'. Childbirth, he urged, was a natural process, which male practitioners from financial motives sought to turn into a 'surgical operation'. Attendance in normal midwifery was the work of women, and should be below the dignity of the professional man. For educated men to submit to the company of nurses and gossips for whole days and nights, merely to assist at the 'humiliating events of parturition', was contrary to decency and common sense.

Midwifery, therefore, should be restored to women, beginning with the womenfolk of surgeons and apothecaries. These practitioners might thereby secure their medical practice against the inroads of their competitors, at the same time establishing 'a respectable maintenance' for their dependants in the event of their own premature death. In addition, the freedom they would gain from unnecessary confinement among the 'gossips' would allow them more time to follow their 'proper vocations'.[25]

In the past the womenfolk of medical practitioners had often practised as midwives, and in France and Germany, where the occupation had higher status, they still did, a considerable number being related to distinguished medical men.[26] In England this appears no longer to have been so,[27] and the British Lying-in Hospital had not received the wife of a surgeon or apothecary as a pupil since 1807. Indeed, to the general practitioner anxious to continue rising in society, Sir Anthony's suggestion must have seemed nothing less than an invitation to social suicide. At a time when uneducated farmers were putting pianos in their parlours and sending their daughters to boarding-school, the medical man with any social pretensions could not be seen allowing his wife to work. Certainly Mr. Gibson, the country surgeon in Mrs. Gaskell's *Wives and Daughters*, would not have made a midwife of his daughter as had Percivall Willughby 170 years before. The place for the womenfolk of men like Gibson was in the drawing-room, waited on as 'ladies'. Indeed, as the young surgeon's wife in Harriet Martineau's *Deerbrook* discovered, even answering the door might lay the gentlewoman open to the charge of 'neglecting appearances'. Should such women face the necessity of earning their own living, the occupation of governess was the only one they could consider, and even this meant degradation in the social scale.[28]

Significantly, Sir Anthony's proposal was greeted with derision by the new medical weekly, the *Lancet*. The *Lancet*'s founder was Thomas Wakley, a young provincial surgeon, who all his life was to champion the interests of the general practitioner against what he saw as the neglect and contempt of the higher echelons of the profession. In a reply which showed how important was the appearance of gentility to the lower ranks of medical men, Wakley thanked God that in England it was 'disreputable' for a husband to require his wife to engage in gainful employment. In Wakley's view it was Sir Anthony's wish to 'degrade' the general practitioner and to ensure that his female relatives would be excluded from 'respectable society'.[29]

But the very achievement of this much sought-after gentility had important psychological consequences for the well-to-do middle-class woman. Shorn of her economic status, she was becoming more and more a mere lady of leisure—the 'pretty fond parasite' described by Thackeray in *Pendennis*, clinging about the sturdy male like the ivy round the oak. Since they were brought up to this role, it is not surprising that these women were considered inferior to men in intellect and courage. Yet if, despite this discouragement, women did essay their talents, even in the genteel field of literature, they were likely to be frowned on as 'unladylike' and 'unwomanly'. It was to escape this censure that Marian Evans and the Brontë sisters published their novels under male pseudonyms.

Such a climate did not foster faith in the capabilities of midwives. Some male practitioners, like Augustus Granville, founder of the Obstetrical Society, saw a place for well-instructed women in the work.[30] There were others, however, who wished to see the midwife totally disappear. Danger in childbirth, they argued, could develop suddenly. Even if women were not precluded from acquiring the necessary anatomical knowledge, as they usually were, they were unfitted by nature for all scientific or mechanical employment. They could therefore never possibly use obstetric instruments with advantage or precision, even if they had presumption enough to try. It followed that it must be safer for the whole of midwifery to be in the hands of men.[31]

A notable proponent of this view was Dr. Samuel Merriman, Physician to the Middlesex Hospital. Despite the fact that his *Difficult Parturition* relates how Mary Dunally, an illiterate Irish midwife, had in 1738 performed the first Caesarian operation to be recorded in the British Isles where both mother and child survived,[32] Merriman would not allow that any midwife had ever made any contribution to the development of the art. Furthermore, he denied that either Elizabeth Nihell or Margaret Stephen had actually written the books published in their names. Mrs. Nihell's, he claimed, was 'said' to have been written by her husband, and Margaret Stephen's by Philip Thicknesse,[33] though how Thicknesse, a journalist, would have been capable of writing a competent midwifery text-book (especially as in 1795 he had been dead three years) Merriman does not say. Small wonder, then that one opponent of male practice protested that in his experience the 'greatest slanders against the moral and intellectual characters of women have been uttered by practitioners of midwifery'.[34]

Sir Anthony Carlisle was not alone in his outspoken objections to the Obstetrical Society's proposals for the institution of formal qualifications for men-midwives. Similar reactions came from the *Examiner* newspaper and the *Monthly Review*, an indication of the opposition which still existed among the general public, and the Radical Tory William Cobbett, looking nostalgically to times past, included a condemnation of man-midwifery in his *Advice to Young*

Men. The affair also gave rise to a crop of pamphlets with the usual sensationalist titles before the accoucheur was denounced both as a 'filthy nondescript' and as a full-time lecher, always ready to use his instruments to save his time and increase his fees.[35] In short, he was nothing but an unprincipled adventurer, ever ready to advance his interests by dishonesty in his own practice and the slander of midwives in theirs.[36]

The columns of the *Lancet* provided an ideal vehicle for the defenders of male practice to return the attack, an exercise in which they had the journal's whole-hearted support. In an oblique reference to the private lying-in homes for the unmarried mother and the prostitute, the *Lancet* asserted that more debauchery was brought about by the 'few female practitioners' in town than could possibly be effected by 'hundreds of lecherous male ones'.[37]

Defending themselves against allegations of a fatal abuse of instruments, accoucheurs pointed to the considerable fall in still-birth and maternal death-rates shown in the London Bills of Mortality since the advent of the male practitioner.[38] This argument was, however, of doubtful validity, since the basis for an accurate assessment of the results of male and female practice did not exist. In the eighteenth century the London Bills provided a very deficient record, both of births and deaths, and during that time there had also been considerable improvement in the provision of trained midwives to the London poor. Moreover, the comparison between mortality rates over so long a period of time ignored the possibility of change in other factors affecting the health and welfare of child-bearing women. Certainly, the abuse of instruments was still common enough to attract the strictures of leading practitioners, and one of these, James Blundell of Guy's, observed that some men seemed to suffer from 'a sort of instinctive impulse to put the lever and the forceps into the vagina'.[39]

Not all opponents of male practice were necessarily champions of female abilities. Sir Henry Halford and Sir Anthony Carlisle, for example, regarded attendance on childbirth as a relatively simple matter not worth the attention of the professional man. Others, while agreeing that midwifery was not generally as complicated as accoucheurs made it out to be, nevertheless recognized the need for thorough and extensive study of the subject. In their view women were quite as capable of midwifery as men, and it was only because their instruction had not kept pace with men's that the contrary notion had arisen.[40] Yet there were enough outstanding midwives whose careers had given powerful proof of female ability and intelligence. A well-known example was Mrs. Ann Newby, Matron of the City of London Lying-in Hospital, who in 1803 had been awarded a gold medal by the Royal Humane Society for saving the lives of over 500 apparently stillborn infants.[41]

But there was another pressing reason why the trend to man-midwifery should be halted. The erosion of women's employment opportunities, which had so alarmed Elizabeth Nihell in 1760 had by now proceeded much further. In 1804 it had attracted the attention of the Clapham Evangelicals, who, commenting on the connection between prostitution and the want of work for women, had set up a Ladies' Committee for Promoting the Education and Employment of the Female Poor. Not only were women entirely excluded from many occupations, the Committee pointed out, but in some which were properly theirs they were 'grievously and unjustly' intruded on by men. If only these traditional employments could be regained from the male 'aggressor', 'millions who might otherwise have sunk in misery and vice might live innocent and happy'.[42] However an attempt shortly afterwards to promote the 'Encouragement and Instruction of Female Midwives' through the foundation in St. George's Fields, London, of a new out-door lying-in charity, the 'British Ladies' Institution', appears to have made little impact, and was probably short-lived.[43]

However, it was the problem of the middle-class woman in need of employment and in particular of the middle-class *girl*, which concerned the pro-midwife pamphleteers of the 1820s. Since 1801, when the first Census was taken, the figures had shown an increasing number of 'surplus' women within the population, and the problem of women's employment had figured largely in the writings of Mary Wollstonecraft and other contemporary advocates of women's rights.[44] Significantly, at the turn of the century, the British Lying-in Hospital had broken with the ancient tradition which required midwives to be married and mothers, and had begun to admit single women as pupils. However, as in the case of the Hôtel-Dieu in Paris where this concession had also been made, it is likely that these were daughters of midwives already in practice.

Similarly, the defenders of the midwife were, for the first time, advocating midwifery as an occupation for *single* women, and their pamphlets outlined the plight of the thousands of 'young females', 'discreetly' brought up and educated, who through a reversal of family fortunes were thrown on their own resources onto a market already over-stocked with unskilled female labour. For want of an alternative, they warned their readers, many of these gentlewomen were forced into prostitution, facing the possibility of misery, disease and premature death. Yet if the legislature could be prevailed upon to provide for the instruction of such women as midwives—if necessary at public expense—not only would they thereby be enabled to live in honest independence, but through the competition of educated women, man-midwifery itself would disappear.[45]

For some advocates of female practice, however, this proposal did not go far enough. The instruction of women pupils, urged a writer to the *Examiner* in 1827, should not stop short at midwifery, but include the study of all the diseases peculiar to women. 'How many myriads of young and shrinking females,' he demanded, 'have been consumed by diseases which delicacy compelled them to conceal from a man, but which they might readily have submitted to a physician of their sex?' Decency and utility equally demanded a change in this custom, and a subscription for the establishment of a 'Female College' for this purpose should be opened forthwith.[46]

It was to be over thirty years before such a College was finally set up. Practical results did follow, however, with the foundation around 1830 in the West End of London of a new 'British Ladies' Lying-in Institution', established under the patronage of Sir Anthony Carlisle, and of several duchesses, including the Duchess of Kent, mother of the Princess Victoria. The Institution's aim was to provide well-trained women, not only for charitable attendance on the poor, but also for private practice among the rich, and it was for this reason that it was established in the fashionable district of Mayfair. Furthermore, as with the larger outdoor-charities its midwives received supervision and instruction, given, however, not by a male practitioner but, in the words of its Prospectus, by its 'Consulting Midwife, Mrs. C. M. Beale, professional attendant to the original patronesses'.[47]

The Charity continued with these arrangements for some years, but by 1858 the 'Consulting Midwife' had been replaced by a 'Surgeon-Accoucheur', and its midwives were henceforward subordinate to men. Like other charities employing midwives, the Ladies' Lying-in Institution had made some contribution to halting the decline in the status of the occupation, but as a venture which aimed at restoring the whole practice to women it had been a dismal failure.

In the meantime there had been another development in the training of women in this field which, however, ran counter to the proposals of those seeking the reinstatement of the midwife. This was the establishment in 1826 by the British Lying-in Hospital of courses for 'monthly' nurses,[48] women who would nurse the mother during the lying-in period, but who (officially at least) were not supposed to deliver the child. For some years now, accoucheurs had been complaining of the lack of competent women to watch labours for them and call them in time for the birth. A good nurse, they urged, was essential in such families as were 'worth attending',[49] and would save the doctor hours of waiting at the bedside without the loss of his fee. Indeed, for the woman who had to earn a living, monthly nursing, in former times an occupation of lower standing than the higher levels of midwifery, might now appear a more lucrative and less arduous employment than independent practice as a midwife, with sole responsibility for the life and health of mother and infant, and increasingly confined to work among the poor. Certainly by the forties and fifties the British Lying-in Hospital was training over three times as many monthly nurses as midwives.

At the same time there had been yet another significant departure from earlier training policy at the hospital. Since their early days, both the British and City of London Hospitals, unlike the other London lying-in hospitals, had taken no male pupils. But in 1831 the British Hospital had changed its policy on this point, and by the 1840s was training as many medical students as midwives. The Governors of the City of London Hospital, however, though repeatedly requested by their medical staff to admit men, resolutely refused to take this step.[50]

The comparative lack of provision for midwife training in England was the subject of outspoken comment by Dr. William Farr, Statistical Superintendent of the newly created Registrar-General's Office, in his report for 1841. With the registration of births and deaths under the 1836 Act, national statistics of maternal mortality were at last available. These showed that over 3,000 mothers (nearly six per thousand registered births) died each year, many as a result of puerperal fever communicated by medical men or midwives attending the birth. It was Dr. Farr's view that if Britain had well-educated and instructed midwives, this toll might be greatly reduced, and many women might be saved from permanent disablement. At the same time a useful occupation would be thrown open to women, who, Farr pointed out to his readers, had few sources of profitable employment.[51]

By contrast with England, several of the principal continental countries now had national schemes for instruction and regulation of midwives.[52] A few years after the opening of the new School for Midwives at the Paris Maternité in 1802, the Prussian government had set up a similar school in Berlin. Admission to this institution continued to be much sought after, preference being given to wives of officials and doctors in the government's service, and by 1837 over 11,000 midwives had been turned out by this and similar government schools in the provinces.[53]

The defenders of the English midwife might well deplore her condition compared with that of her continental counterpart. France had produced a number of distinguished midwives, of whom Mme

Lachapelle, author of the outstanding *Pratique d'Accouchements* (1821-5), and Mme Boivin, whose many medical honours included a doctorate from the University of Marburg, were the most famous. A similar distinction had been conferred by the University of Giessen on the German midwife, Regina von Siebold, whose daughter Charlotte later obtained a regular doctorate at the same university. It was Charlotte who travelled to England in 1819 and delivered the infant Princess Victoria, and, on returning to Germany, Victoria's cousin and future Consort, Prince Albert of Saxe-Coburg Gotha.

But despite his undisguised admiration of State-controlled schools for midwives in France and Prussia, Farr conceded that it would be 'folly' to expect the British, with the 'undoubted difference' in their manners and institutions, to establish such a system.[54] One factor adverse to such a development was the traditional British mistrust of any extension of government powers, particularly those of central government, shown so clearly in the hostility which was to hamper and finally emasculate Chadwick's Board of Health. Another was the new fear of over-population which had accompanied the rapid rise in numbers since 1800, and it was these Malthusian anxieties which had largely inspired the repressive régime for the management of the destitute poor established under the New Poor Law of 1834. Yet over the past ten years, Government had shown an increased willingness to countenance State compulsion and provision in health matters, as demonstrated by the Act for the registration of births, marriages and deaths, the 1833 Factory Act, and, most remarkable of all, the institution in 1840 of a nation-wide State-provided vaccination service, free and open to all, regardless of means.

Seeking a cause for the relative lack of provision for midwife training in England, Farr himself was inclined to attribute this to 'national delicacy' in matters of this kind.[55] This 'delicacy' was a relatively recent development, and was largely the achievement of the 'Evangelical' religious movement which in the space of a few decades had completely bowdlerized the language and literature of 'respectable' society.[56] It was not just that matters of sex and reproduction might be mentioned only in the obliquest manner; the taboo extended to the sexual denominations of animals, and even to the names of underwear, for which must now be substituted newly invented euphemisms and circumlocutions. The word 'midwife', too, had lost caste, and in *Martin Chuzzlewit* (1844) Dickens chooses to describe Mrs. Gamp as a 'monthly nurse', almost apologizing for her outspoken signboard, which boldly proclaimed her a 'Midwife'.

This prudery particularly affected women. The range of literature available to girls was severely restricted, and, as Bessie Rayner

Parkes, a leading figure in the subsequent campaign for women's education was to observe, girls were kept away from Chaucer, Dryden, Jonson and Fielding, 'as from the plague or cholera'.[57] *Tom Jones*, if read at all, was 'a man's book',[58] and, as Thackeray complained in his introduction to *Pendennis*, no writer since Fielding's death might depict life as it really was without offending his lady readers and so affecting his sales. In these circumstances it was increasingly difficult for the genteel woman of the 'respectable' classes even to consider midwifery as an occupation, however great her need of a livelihood.

Notions of delicacy were also invoked to keep the husband from the lying-in room. In a letter to the *Lancet* occasioned by newspaper reports of the Prince Consort's presence at the birth of the Prince of Wales, a 'Country Doctor' protested against such 'intrusion' by husbands, which offended against his 'old fashioned notions of delicacy and propriety'. He himself had had two cases of patients from London, whose husbands, despite all his efforts to discourage them by repeated 'black looks', had remained in the lying-in room. 'Country Doctor' was supported in his condemnation of this new upper-class fashion by a number of correspondents who agreed that it was 'highly indelicate', 'indecent, unbecoming, and unnecessary', and 'contrary to nature'. Others, however, disagreed. Appeals to delicacy at such a time, declared one, were 'unworthy of a liberal profession'. Many wives would welcome their husbands' support and sympathy in their ordeal; moreover, if husbands actually *saw* what went on at the birth, any suspicions about the doings of the accoucheur in the lying-in room, and the reserve with which he was often subsequently regarded, would disappear.[59]

A lay correspondent, on the other hand, saw the question in a different light. Why, he asked, was it an indelicate intrusion for the husband to be present, but acceptable for the accoucheur—a man and a stranger? Predictably, his suggestion that the employment of properly educated midwives would remove the need for this greater indelicacy provoked the standard hostile response. Men had more moral courage than women, wrote one reader. Boys, wrote another, learnt more about mechanical forces from their rough and destructive play with toys and furniture than girls could ever do from nursing dolls: females were thus 'very unlikely to prove ingenious in any really mechanical operation, which midwifery is'. The *Lancet* had the last word. Taking its usual anti-midwife and, indeed, anti-feminist line, the journal reassured its readers that

With regard to the advocacy of midwives, the women of England are, happily for her sons [presumably, the medical profession] wholly deficient both in the moral and physical organisation necessary for performing the duties of that most responsible office.[60]

Indeed the rashness and incompetence of ignorant midwives was a continuing theme in the medical journals which under the title of 'Midwives' Midwifery' regularly included reports of childbirth fatalities where midwives had been in attendance. The midwife might have torn out the patient's womb, pulled the child's body from its head, or perpetrated lesser, but nevertheless permanent, injuries on both mother or child. However, the journals also carried stories of male practitioners who in their ignorance had actually cut out the womb, or part of the intestines, with scissors or knife.[61] Some of these—graphically referred to by the *London Medical Gazette* as 'disembowelling accoucheurs'—were regularly qualified men; others, often chemists, merely passed as such. The publicity which these cases received led to demands that the current Government Bill for the regulation of medicine should require that in future all qualified medical men should hold a qualification in midwifery, and that unqualified midwifery practice, by men *or* women, should be declared illegal. Yet, complained the *Gazette*, because of exaggerated notions of the importance of individual liberty, all the Government did was to print the mortality statistics for the information of the survivors.[62]

But far from inclining towards prohibition of unqualified practice, Parliament was moving steadily away from it. Many medical men were critical of the way in which the Society of Apothecaries had exercised the prohibitory powers granted under the 1815 Act, complaining that it was quicker to prosecute well-qualified Irish and Scottish doctors than the ignorant and dangerous quack.[63] Significantly, in the chemists' registration Act of 1852, Parliament had merely applied the Free Trade principle of distinguishing the qualified practitioner from the unqualified, leaving the public to choose between them. Finally, in 1858, after various Bills for the regulation of the medical profession had been intermittently before Parliament for nearly twenty years, the successful Government measure of that year adopted the same principle.

Thus the Act made no provision for penalizing unqualified practice. Instead, it established a system for the registration of practitioners holding qualifications from degree- and diploma-granting bodies recognized by the new General Council for Medical Education and Registration set up under the Act. It did nothing about midwives, and nothing, moreover, to require future medical practitioners admitted to the Register to qualify themselves in midwifery, an omission which gave legal confirmation to the still current view that this specialty was not really part of medicine.[64] Further, because the Universities and corporations admitted only men to their examination, the Act appeared to put the final seal on the exclusion of women from the profession.

Despite the Act's failure to recognize midwifery as an integral part of medicine, its status as an occupation for medical men had risen considerably since the efforts of the short-lived Obstetrical Society thirty years before. Several medical examining bodies now required midwifery to be in the curriculum, and some were examining in it.[65] In 1852 the College of Surgeons had finally set up a Midwifery Licence for those wishing to gain such a qualification, and had also abandoned the bye-law which barred the election of practitioners of midwifery to its Council. This last step had been taken a few years earlier by the College of Physicians, and already several distinguished 'obstetricians' (as they were now beginning to call themselves) had been raised to the dignity of Fellows of that body.

But there was still a long way to go to secure the acceptance of midwifery on an equal footing with other branches of medicine. It was to work for this recognition that a few months after the passage of the Medical Act a group of London obstetricians joined together to form a new Obstetrical Society. The purpose of the Society, membership of which was to be open to any registered medical practitioner, was to establish a forum for the scientific discussion of obstetrics, and thus to provide for this branch what the numerous other medical societies provided for medicine and surgery.

The subject of midwives was raised at the Society's first meeting by a founder member, Dr. C. F. H. Routh. Dr. Routh felt strongly that in working towards an improvement in obstetric practice the Society should not lose sight of the 'political element', and that legislation for midwife regulation should also figure among its objects.[66] This view does not seem to have met with much response from the Society's members, however. Among specialist obstetricians there were those who held that the specialty would never take its rightful place while midwives still existed, and many general practitioners, far from wishing to see midwives trained and regulated, looked forward to the day when they could be legally excluded from practice. Indeed, though he later moderated his opinions,[67] such views had been forcibly expressed some years before by the Society's principal founder, Dr. Tyler Smith, when Lecturer in Midwifery at the Hunterian School of Medicine. 'All midwives are a mistake', Smith had told his students, and it should be the steady aim of every obstetric practitioner to discourage their employment. The office of midwife should be abolished, and the very word 'midwifery' done away with on account of its derivation.[68]

Tyler Smith had accompanied this outburst with an onslaught on lying-in charities for their training and employment of midwives. It was only because midwives were 'legitimised' and 'diplomatised' by these institutions, he complained, that they were preserved to compete with the general practitioner in the lower walks of practice and in the Poor Law Medical Service. Singling out the Royal Maternity Charity as the oldest and largest of its kind, Smith launched a bitter attack on this institution. For it to be publicly admitted that parturient women should be attended by midwives, however well instructed, was 'degrading' to the obstetric branch of medicine. Moreover, it was questionable charity to supply to the poor what would not be considered good enough for the rich. Despite its 'glowing' annual reports, the Charity's practice *must* be less safe than if it employed 'educated accoucheurs' for all its cases.[69]

A few years later, in 1854, on the occasion of a dispute among the Charity's medical staff, the *Lancet* itself had taken up this cry, castigating the Charity for its 'inhumanity' in employing midwives. The Charity's Governors promptly returned the *Lancet*'s fire. For the century of its existence, they pointed out, the organization had assisted over 400,000 women in childbirth, with proportionately lower mortality than under any other system in use by any similar institution. Its midwives constituted a class of well-instructed matrons, trained by one of its own physicians. Besides serving the Charity's patients, they satisfied a demand from other women in the neighbourhood who, either from pecuniary considerations, or from choice alone, 'gladly' resorted to midwives. Midwives had always formed an integral part of the Royal Maternity Charity and were 'a most valuable medium for carrying out its benevolent designs'.[70]

Indeed, on the question of the relative safety of the Charity's practice, its critics were on uncertain ground. The Charity's statistics, published by the eminent obstetricians who supervised and participated in its work, showed that although it served poor working-class women, often living in unhealthy conditions, its maternal death-rate was lower than the Registrar-General's figure for the country at large.[71] Over the years, together with other charities run on similar lines, the Charity was also to show a lower rate than that in the practice of some of the 'educated accoucheurs' themselves, who however practised largely among the better-off.

In common with other practitioners in whom the wish was father to the thought, Dr. Tyler Smith had also claimed that midwife attendance was the exception rather than the rule.[72] But although this was now probably true of the West End of London and other affluent areas, over the country at large the majority of births were still attended by women.[73] However, because most midwives practised on a part-time basis, the Census returns consistently underestimated their numbers.[74]

The better trained midwives, as always, were to be found in the larger towns. Some of them were in salaried posts in hospitals or workhouse infirmaries where they would have been paid £30 to £40 per annum, plus board and lodging, that is, a salary equivalent to that generally received by an upper servant or a governess. Others were employed on the out-door staff of Unions, hospitals, or other charities; although the fees were generally not more than 5s. for Poor Law cases and often less for charity work, particularly in the provinces, such appointments conferred a respectability on the holder which gave her a recognized advantage in competition for private practice.

In cities, established midwives working for well-known charities and engaging in private practice appear to have made an income of 25s. to £2.10s. per week, an amount comparable with that earned by the skilled working man or the humbler clerk or teacher.[75] Some of the more experienced midwives, like Mrs. Catherine Jones, who had been for many years on the out-door staff of Queen Charlotte's Hospital, were able to charge from 15s. to four guineas in their private practice.[76] If, like Mrs. Mate, midwife to the Islington Union and to a number of local charities, they took on a large number of cases, they might make a very comfortable living compared with the few shillings a week to be had from most employments open to married women working from home.[77] The more fortunate of such midwives would be sought out by those of the wealthier classes who still preferred female attendance. According to the pro-midwife pamphlet The Accoucheur, the private practice of Mrs. Elizabeth Mate would 'suprise' everyone, while 'a lady at the Court End of London' regularly received fees of ten guineas, or thirty, when, as frequently happened, she attended the aristocracy.

But the general picture was one of decline. In some areas midwives might attend the wives of small tradesmen or farmers, but in others their clientele consisted only of the class just above paupers, and here such women eked out a poor living with other humble work, like washing or charing. In some more affluent districts they might have hardly any cases at all. Their employment under the Poor Law was also decreasing; in some Unions they were no longer employed, either for out-door cases, or, as in the majority of the Metropolitan Unions, in the workhouse wards. However, in the workhouse the absence of a midwife meant that it was often the unqualified nurse who actually delivered the child, rather than the doctor whose proper responsibility it was.[78]

As always, most women practising as midwives had no training at all. Occasionally a general practitioner living in a sparsely populated area might give some instruction to local women, in order that they might attend those whose small fees would not reimburse him for hours spent travelling over long distances and waiting in humble cottages.[79] Lying-in hospitals and charities still took midwife pupils, but the number trained was small. The greatest contribution to training was probably being made by St. Mary's Hospital, Manchester, which was to boast that it had trained more midwives even than the Rotunda in Dublin.[80]

The general tendency, however, seems to have been against the training of midwives. When Professor Burden tried to start this in the mid-1850s at Queen's Hospital, Belfast, he met with much opposition, the Ladies' Committee of that institution objecting that it was impossible that a woman could need, or profit from, the proposed instruction. In the London hospitals at this period, midwife training was certainly declining. The British Lying-in Hospital, which a hundred years before had prided itself on this aspect of its work for the public, now had hardly any midwife pupils at all. Though since 1845 it had ceased to take medical students, the women it was now instructing were predominantly monthly nurses whose training benefited only the well-to-do who could afford to employ them, and the better-off doctors, whose time they saved.

Thus it was that by the 1850s the situation foreseen by Elizabeth Nihell a hundred years before had arrived. Despite repeated proposals for the rehabilitation and regulation of midwives, none of these had come to fruition, and now the stigma attaching to the occupation was such that educated entrants to it were rare indeed.[81] It was not the dignified professionalism of women like Margaret Stephen which the word 'midwife' conjured up in the minds of the middle classes from whom leading midwives had once been recruited. Instead, there arose the sinister image of 'Mother Midnight', or, at the very least, the garrulous, tippling, and distinctly unprofessional figure of Dickens' Sairey Gamp. Forty years before, in 1817, the family of an old Norwich midwife, Mrs. Phoebe Crewe, had proudly recorded on her gravestone her forty years' work in this calling.[82] Now, the word 'midwife' itself was hardly respectable, and Sairey's continuing celebrity was to eclipse all the skilled, sober, dedicated, and educated women who had preceded her.

By contrast, the social standing of her male rival, the general practitioner, had been rising steadily, and the specialty of obstetrics, though not yet officially recognized as part of medicine, had at least been accorded acceptance by the medical Establishment. At the same time, chemists and dentists, who, like midwives, shared their field with the medical profession, were also making rapid strides towards professional status. Like medical practitioners, both these categories had for some years now possessed their own nationally based professional organizations and their own professional journals. The chemists' professional body, the Pharmaceutical Society, had obtained State registration for duly qualified chemists in 1852, six years before the Medical Act, and in 1859 the specialty of dentistry had been officially recognized with the institution by the Royal College of Surgeons of a Licence in Dental Surgery.

With midwives things were very different. There were no midwives' societies, and no midwives' journals, and, since the publication in 1797 of Martha Mears' *Pupil of Nature*, no midwifery work published by a midwife. Unlike Mrs. Hester Shaw and her colleagues of two hundred years before, those midwives who were educated enough and respectable enough to wish to improve the status of their occupation were too few and too weak to join together to defend or further their interests. Most midwives had to work very long hours to make even an adequate living, and few could have had the education or the leisure necessary to organize themselves for the improvement of the general body. Indeed, at a time when in the public eye the lot of the woman who sought self-advancement was condemnation and ridicule, and the subject of midwifery could not be mentioned in polite female society, any attempt on the part of a midwife to set on foot such a venture would not only have required more than ordinary courage but would certainly have met with failure.

In these circumstances, if the deterioration in the position of English midwives was ever to be halted, it was inevitable that the initiative would have to come from outside their ranks. Without such external help, the downward trend would continue, until, as their enemies confidently hoped and expected, a time would arrive when what had traditionally been a woman's employment would become a virtual monopoly of the all-male medical profession. If this happened, there would be two important consequences to women as a sex. First, those needing to work would no longer have the chance of earning their living in an occupation which for centuries had been the refuge of the unsupported wife or widow. Second, whatever their feelings of modesty in this situation, all women seeking skilled assistance in childbirth would henceforth be forced to put themselves into the hands of men.

CHAPTER FOUR

The Turn of the Tide

In 1760 the midwife Elizabeth Nihell had deplored the general lack of work for women and had pointed to the steady loss of traditional female occupations to men. As already mentioned, this loss was the result of the combination of a number of factors, all related to the increasing industrialization and growing wealth of society. Over the next hundred years this process was to continue without interruption, bringing with it an inevitable worsening of women's economic and social position relative to that of men.

This was not merely a question of a few specialized employments like midwifery or hair-dressing, however. During this time women were also largely excluded, both at managerial and counter level, from the world of business. Industrialization had brought new independence to the women who worked in the factories, but had made it harder for mothers of young children to earn money. For middle-class women who had to support themselves the loss of opportunities for work was equally, if not more, serious. Increasing emphasis on the maintenance of genteel appearances had barred to gentlewomen many of their traditional employments, at the same time breeding a contempt for those whom adversity forced to earn their own bread. Indeed, it is probably no exaggeration to say that in the mid-nineteenth century the circumstances of the unsupported gentlewoman were worse than at any time before or since.[1]

Yet women's need for work was in fact much greater than when Elizabeth Nihell wrote a hundred years before. Ever since the first census in 1801 the returns had shown an excess of women over men which rose steadily with each decade. By 1851 there were over a quarter of a million more women than men in the 20–40 age-group; in consequence, a large number of women had to remain single all their lives. Despite the Victorian idealization of home-making as a woman's proper sphere, these 'redundant' or 'superfluous' women were forced, together with many widows and deserted wives, to earn their own living.

The actual proportion of women working at this period is difficult to discover. The 1851 Census Report itself gave a quarter of wives and two-thirds of widows as gainfully occupied. Others have put the proportion of all women working at this time at about a quarter, or at nearly a third.[2] However, when account is taken of the general under-recording of women's part-time work, it seems more than likely that these are conservative estimates.

For lower-class women the largest single occupation was domestic service which, though expanding, was generally unsuitable for the woman with dependent children. Other principal employments were factory or field work, the domestic industries, or the grinding, unhealthy toil in dress-making, millinery, or 'slopwork'—the cheap plain sewing done at home. Many workers in the needle trades could not earn even the barest subsistence, and drifted in and out of the ranks of the prostitutes who walked the streets of London and other great cities.[3] Prostitution itself was thought to be growing, and under the euphemistic title of the 'Social Evil' was increasingly attracting public attention.[4]

The choice facing middle-class women seeking work was even more restricted. A few gifted and fortunate ones, like Harriet Martineau, or Lady Blessington, made a living by journalism and literature, but most turned to the only respectable alternative open to them—the overstocked and poorly paid occupation of governess. Though the more general adoption of the upper-class custom of educating daughters at home had greatly enlarged the demand for governesses, the same aspirations to gentility had also added to the supply. In the past many poor clergymen's daughters, like Fielding's Mrs. Slip-Slop in *Joseph Andrews*, had been content to work as housekeepers or ladies' maids, or keep a small shop. Now they became governesses, as did the daughters of ambitious farmers and tradesmen who hoped thereby to advance their social position.[5]

In 1851 the Census recorded over 21,000 women working as governesses. Pay varied: a few received an annual salary of £100 or more, but the usual rate was £35 (the wage of an upper servant in a well-to-do household) and many were paid much less.[6] Low pay was only part of the story, however. Removed socially from the servants by her superior pretensions, often slighted by the family and bullied by the children, a governess commonly led a dreary existence, her loneliness further aggravated by her employer's reluctance to allow her to receive visitors or make new friends.[7] Worse still, after spending the greater part of their lives in this isolation, many governesses found themselves penniless in old age,[8] and some were forced to end their days in the pauper uniform of the workhouse —a doubly cruel degradation to middle-class women brought up to regard the deterrent regime of the Poor Law as a just reward for improvidence and vice.

The difficulties of the unsupported gentlewoman had been stressed by the defenders of the midwife over and over again since the 1790s. Now, through the publicity given to the plight of the governess, it had at last begun to engage the active and continuing attention of the philanthropically disposed. In 1843 the Governesses' Benevolent Institution, which aimed to succour impoverished governesses, was founded by the Christian Socialist clergyman, F. D. Maurice, and a few years later efforts were set in hand to enable gentlewomen to emigrate to the colonies. But if middle-class girls were to compete more effectively in the governess market they had to receive better education than the faulty and limited instruction generally open to them. It was to provide this that in 1848 Maurice, together with a fellow Christian Socialist, the Reverend Charles Kingsley, established Queen's College for Women in Harley Street. Among the students during the school's earlier years were Frances Buss and Dorothea Beale, themselves to play an important part in girls' education, and Sophia Jex-Blake, one of the pioneers of women's admission to the medical profession. Queen's was followed shortly afterwards by Bedford College for Ladies (1849), North London Collegiate School (1850), and Cheltenham Ladies' College (1853). These foundations did more than provide girls with much needed secondary education; they also paved the way for the entry of the next generation of girls to higher education. This came, not without considerable efforts on the part of the women's movement and a determined fight on that of the opposition, with the admission of women in 1878 to the degrees of the University of London and within the next twenty years to the examinations of Oxford and Cambridge.

Women suffered from other economic disabilities, however, besides lack of employment or the education to fit them for it. One was the legal inability of married women to own property. In the eyes of the law, a married woman had the legal and contractual status of a minor, and all her possessions, including her earnings, were her husband's—even if he had deserted her and no longer maintained her. In 1855 this question was taken up by a group of upper middle-class women led by Barbara, the twenty-five-year-old daughter of the Unitarian Radical M.P., Benjamin Leigh Smith. Two years later, with the aid of the Law Amendment Society, a Bill to remove these disabilities was introduced into Parliament. The Bill failed, however, the reformers' only consolation being the enactment the same year of the Matrimonial Causes Act, which allowed deserted or legally separated wives to keep their own earnings. It was not until 1883 that married women gained full control over their property.

Yet despite this disappointment, the campaign for the Bill had brought great gains to the cause of women's rights. To obtain support for the Bill Barbara Leigh Smith had assembled a committee of women to collect signatures for a petition in its favour and it was from this first concerted political action that an entirely new phenomenon—a movement for the advancement of women's rights —may be said to have originated. Thus far, efforts to improve the condition of women had been sporadic and isolated. Now, however, they were to coalesce into a national women's movement committed to fight for the removal of legal disabilities, for entry to higher education and the professions, and for the Parliamentary and local franchise. Moreover, it was a movement in which women themselves were to play a leading and vocal part.[9]

Hitherto a very small number of women had had any experience of political organization. Though a few, like the dedicated social reformer and feminist Josephine Butler, had been brought up in households where political activity on behalf of causes like the abolition of slavery and the repeal of the Corn Laws was part of daily life, in general the public life of women had been limited to the management of parish charities. However, the rapid growth of the middle classes over the past half century had produced an increasing number of women with time to devote to such work, and a corresponding increase in the philanthropic organizations founded and run by them. It was a mark of women's improved status, the *Lancet* stated proudly in 1857, that there was not a town in the kingdom which did not have its lying-in society, female school, visiting association, nursing institute, and many other charitable organizations exclusively managed by the 'gentler sex'.[10] But although these 'ladies' societies' were generally confined to the parish level, already there were women like Elizabeth Fry, the prison reformer, and Mary Carpenter, notable for her work on behalf of juvenile delinquents, who had achieved a national reputation. As the century wore on there were to be more such figures whose achievements, along with those of the political activists of the new women's movement, were to go a long way towards changing the public image of women as inevitably dependent and subordinate members of society.

But the path of the women's movement was far from easy. Contempt and ridicule were heaped upon its members by opponents —women as well as men—who objected that the emancipated woman would lose her 'essential' feminine nature. A typical and persistent critic was the *Saturday Review* which, taking the lordly standpoint of the 'higher sex', never missed a chance of deriding the 'petticoat rebellion' and its 'strong-minded' advocates of woman's rights. The *Review* was unimpressed by the disabilities of married women, or the need of unsupported women for gainful employment, arguing that any increase in the number of women working would only reduce the employment open to men. Whatever their circumstances, women should not be encouraged to seek economic independence, lest the whole sex develop a distaste for the 'tedious duties' of marriage. 'Married life', the *Review* maintained in 1859,

> is a woman's profession . . . of course, by not getting a husband, or losing him, she may find that she is without resources. All that can be said of her is, she has failed in business, and no social reform can prevent such failures.[11]

In 1859 an attempt was made to help women seeking employment, when the growing group of lady reformers, members of the new women's movement, founded a Society for Promoting the Employment of Women. The Society's offices were at 19, Langham Place, the home of the movement's new periodical, the *Englishwoman's Journal*. The chief aim of the Society was to expand employment for women of the lower middle classes whose competition for the work of governess they considered to be depressing the market, and among the occupations advocated in the Society's annual reports were law copying, clerical work, book-keeping, telegraphy, shoe-making and cookery. The traditional woman's calling of midwifery was not mentioned, however—a significant testimony to the low esteem in which the midwife was now generally held. Yet nursing, also an employment in which most of the workers were poor and uneducated[12]—Sairey Gamp, it must be remembered, was a sick nurse as well as a midwife—was nevertheless included. However, this 'noble profession' was only considered suitable for 'grave earnest women, past their first youth, whose love of gaiety and amusement has subsided', and who possessed strong nerves and superior intelligence.[13]

This new higher status of nursing was largely the consequence of the remarkable achievements of Miss Florence Nightingale in the recent Crimean War. The handsome, witty and talented daughter of a rich upper-class family, Florence had refused more than one eligible suitor, rejecting marriage in order to devote herself to the great task of hospital reform for which she was convinced God had destined her. Finally, at the age of thirty-one, and in the teeth of family opposition, she took the unconventional step for a young woman of her social rank of going to work as a nurse at the Kaiserswerth Institute near Düsseldorf. Expected by her family to resume her filial duties on her return, she had to face a long and agonizing struggle before she at last broke free to follow an independent life. In 1853 she was offered the post of Superintendent in a small nursing home in London, the Institution for the Care of Sick Gentlewomen in Distressed Circumstances. It was from there, late in 1854, that she went to Scutari at the invitation of her friend and fellow reformer Sidney Herbert, Secretary of State for War, to organize the nursing of British soldiers.

Miss Nightingale and her nurses had suffered great hardship, but her political skill, her unrivalled powers of organization, and above all her indomitable spirit, had triumphed over the bungling of Army officials and the obstruction of medical staff to bring order out of chaos and save hundreds of lives. On her return to England she was to devote the rest of her long life to the training of nurses, the reform of hospital administration, and the improvement of services to the British soldier throughout the Empire.

Miss Nightingale's achievements were to be of especial significance to women. Not only did the homage rendered her by a grateful nation represent a powerful challenge to current assumptions of essential feminine incompetence and frailty, but her work for nursing was to have important consequences for women's employment. Hitherto the great body of nurses had been older women from the domestic servant class, and some were undoubtedly of 'low character' and given to drink. Only sisters and matrons had come from a higher level of society, being commonly widows in reduced circumstances who were recruited separately from ordinary nurses.[14] Now Miss Nightingale's own practical example, together with the spirit of dedication which she had brought to the work, were to invest nursing with the sanctity of a religious vocation. As such, nursing could now offer an alternative occupation to women who would otherwise have become governesses, and one which in contrast might lead to real influence and power. Nursing also presented an acceptable avenue of escape from the prison of the Victorian drawing-room —indicted so bitterly by Miss Nightingale herself in her unpublished essay 'Cassandra'[15]—and must have meant a welcome release to many women facing the dreary and stigmatized future of an 'old maid'.

Nursing was also made more attractive to 'respectable' girls by the establishment in 1860 of the Nightingale Nurse Training School at St. Thomas' Hospital, London. The school was run according to plans drawn up by Miss Nightingale herself, and financed from a fund subscribed by a grateful public. Nurse training was already being undertaken in some other institutions, but the social position and influence of Miss Nightingale lent great prestige to the St.

Thomas' School. Not only were her pupil nurses carefully selected and supervised, but their training lasted a whole year, and, like their board and lodging, was free; moreover, although still pupils, they were paid into the bargain. Thus was laid the foundation of the movement which within thirty years was to raise nursing from menial work considered fit at best for house-maids with no special skills, to the level of a respected profession in which gentlewomen could earn their living.[16]

Again, the occupation of nurse was more in tune with current ideas of female propriety than was midwifery. Until the development of district nursing, the 'new' nurse would either live in hospital, under the supervision of the matron, or nurse the well-off and respectable in their own homes. But the private work of the midwife, the nature of which was in any case unmentionable in polite female society, lay usually among the poor, and might bring comparatively little return. To pursue it, a woman had to go out alone at night, something a respectable girl was not allowed to do.[17] Worse still, she had to risk exposure to the coarse language and manners from which it was the aim of every genteel family to shelter its womenfolk. Among the poor, childbirth was still an occasion for generous indulgence by the patient and attendant company in alcoholic refreshment and, as like as not, bawdy humour.[18] It is not surprising that the middle-class feminists of Langham Place, anxious to secure the success of their pioneering venture, did not recommend this occupation to their clients.

It is for her work in the reform of nursing that Miss Nightingale is chiefly remembered. It is less well known, however, that she also cherished an ambition to bring about as great an improvement in the practice and status of midwives. Forcibly struck with the poor provision for midwife instruction in England compared with that on the Continent, she had decided with characteristic determination and energy, to make her own contribution to midwife training by founding her own school. With the financial backing of the Nightingale Fund and the co-operation of King's College Hospital she opened her school in an annexe of the Hospital in 1861. 'In nearly every country but our own,' she wrote to Harriet Martineau, 'there is a Government School for Midwives. I trust that our school may lead the way towards supplying a long felt want in England.'[19]

Miss Nightingale's scheme was to supply trained midwives for work among the rural poor. Suitable village women were sent up as pupils by local clergymen and landowners, returning to serve their own parishes. In recognition of the fact that the small fees they received from this work were insufficient to keep them, the women were generally subsidized by their sponsors. The training lasted six months—longer than that offered elsewhere in the United Kingdom except at the Rotunda in Dublin. But the school aimed to train only limited numbers, and it was Miss Nightingale's hope that, like the Nurse Training School at St. Thomas', it would serve as a model which others would copy throughout the country.[20]

Although the training offered by the school was superior to that available elsewhere in England, Miss Nightingale insisted that outgoing pupils should be certified as 'Midwifery Nurses' rather than 'Midwives'. In contrast to the current medical view, it was her firm opinion that a midwife proper should be capable of dealing with *all* cases including those of difficulty and danger, and her training should not be less than the two years' course available for the higher class of midwives in France.[21]

Unfortunately for Miss Nightingale's plans, there were persistent outbreaks of puerperal fever in the wards of her school (attributed by her to its proximity to the Hospital's post-mortem theatre) and in 1867 she regretfully closed it down. For a long time it was her fond hope that she might open a new school 'under happier sanitary conditions', this time with Government help, and enlarge its scope for the training of more highly educated women as 'fully qualified midwives'.[22] But this hope was never realized. Rehabilitating the midwife was to prove a much more difficult task than up-grading the nurse. The provision of clean, sober and reliable women for nursing in private households was of direct interest to the rich and influential, and to their medical attendants. These were therefore ready to give active support to nursing reform. By contrast the clientele of the midwife consisted mainly of the poor and inarticulate. With her powerful influence in medical and political circles, Miss Nightingale could without doubt have done much for the reinstatement of the midwife. But as it turned out her attention was diverted from midwifery by her commitments in other fields, and this work, though always remaining dear to her heart, was left to others.

Despite the continuing deterioration in the midwife's position, there were still members of the aristocracy and middle classes who resisted the spread of male practice and who refused to follow the fashion in employing a man. The old sensationalist pamphlets denouncing man-midwifery—the work of doctors and other professional men—were still appearing.[23] Occasionally, more restrained pro-midwife opinions found expression in the better-class journals; and in his popular collection of essays, *Horae Subsecivae*, Dr. John Brown, a Fellow of the Edinburgh College of Physicians, showed that opposition to the male practitioner still persisted in the higher ranks of the medical profession.[24] At the same time, revelations by leading obstetricians exposing the lucrative gynaecological quackery currently practised by some of their number furnished their opponents with further ammunition in the continuing battle against man-midwifery.[25]

The champions of the midwife continued to advocate the occupation as suitable for middle-class women who had to earn their living; and in 1859 the author of a new pro-midwife pamphlet, *The Accoucheur*, prefaced it with a warning on the desperate condition in which many such women found themselves:

> You may teach that poor, but beautiful orphan girl morality; but she needs bread, and her needle does not make enough to sustain her, though she plies it almost day and night. The labour market in which she has to compete with others is over-stocked, and the competition is fierce. All this because woman is shut out from much of the work for which her tact and talent, her sympathy and position would fit her. Society has no mercy on her. She could work our telegraphs, serve the counter, act the midwife, supply, at least to her own sex, more than the accomplished physician; but in all those spheres strong men supplant her; and scarcely a choice is left to her in the sphere of honest, independent labour, but to sew in the garret or toil in the fields.[26]

The proposal that women should be admitted to the medical profession had been gaining increasing support in recent years, much of it among the upper and middle classes. In America, where a rear-guard action was also being fought against the encroachments of man-midwifery,[27] a number of women had already qualified as medical practitioners. Elizabeth Blackwell, who had qualified in the State of New York in 1849, had been the first. Now she was in England lecturing on 'Medicine as a Profession for Ladies', and under a once-and-for-all arrangement for resident practitioners holding foreign qualifications was admitted to the new Medical Register. One woman, at least, was officially recognized as qualified for medical practice.

Advocates of the medical woman's cause employed three main arguments. A large number of women, they pointed out, *had* to work, and their exclusion from this occupation ran contrary to the prevailing economic doctrine of Free Trade.[28] Moreover, there were many women in urgent need of medical attention who refused to consult a man or, if they did, could not bring themselves to give him a full account of their more intimate symptoms, or to permit him to make a thorough examination.[29] For these reasons it was imperative that there should be fully qualified female practitioners for women desiring attendance by their own sex. Finally, it was hoped that medical women would take more interest in the diseases of women and children, a department of medicine thought by many not to receive proper attention from the profession.[30]

These were practical considerations. Another important factor was the long-standing belief that male attendance had a corrupting effect on society. It was thus one of the major obstacles to the 'grand moral reform' to which many influential members of the women's movement aspired. One such was Mrs. Josephine Butler, later leader of the campaign against the State regulation of prostitution instituted under the Contagious Diseases Acts of the 1860s, who felt passionately on 'this bitter and awful subject'. In her view male attendance in female complaints was nothing less than a 'profanation' of the 'best and purest feelings' of womankind, which only the 'intrinsically noble and good' could survive without permanent degradation of their moral nature. Mrs. Butler herself had been attended by a midwife at the birth of each of her four children, and declared that she herself and others like her, would risk death 'willingly' rather than be guilty of what was unbearable before God. Women faced this cruel dilemma, she wrote, solely because of the 'tyranny' of the medical profession in denying them the opportunity of consulting fully qualified practitioners of their own sex. In this way the profession had been responsible for inflicting pain and moral injury on 'generation after generation' of women. While this 'wicked custom' persisted, the 'moral renovation' of society could never be fully achieved.[31]

This 'dilemma' against which Mrs. Butler protested so bitterly had been exacerbated by the extreme conditioning in prudery to which middle-class girls had been subjected over the past half century, and which Mrs. Butler herself dignified with the sanction of religion. The ironic result was that if what the *Guardian* newspaper called 'true delicacy' were to be maintained between the sexes,[32] carefully nurtured young gentlewomen would have to take on work which for many years past had been regarded as suitable only for older women of a lower class or for the male sex.

Official medical opinion on the issue of women's entry into medicine had already declared itself in 1856. In that year Miss Jessie Meriton White had applied to the Royal College of Surgeons and to the University of London to know if they would be willing to admit a woman to their examinations. Both had refused, to the amusement of the *British Medical Journal*, which considered the whole question a great joke.[33] Significantly, there were lay critics who viewed the matter in a different light, charging these two bodies with displaying the 'same sordid spirit of monopoly' as the Army medical staff who had recently attempted to thwart Florence Nightingale in the Crimea.[34]

Not all medical men were opposed to the idea, however, and some distinguished practitioners were to be numbered among its supporters. But in general the reaction of the profession was hostile. Denying that the question was one of general interest or necessity, the *Lancet* dismissed the campaign as merely a 'morbid' agitation on the part of a few misguided ladies who, with a contrariness characteristic of their sex, sought to open up to women the one profession for which they were least suited. Even if it could be granted that women were equal to men in intellect and 'decision of character'—and were not women in every civilized country losing their old field of midwifery to men?—the divinely ordained physical disqualifications entailed in their duties as wives and mothers unfitted them for medical practice. Yet the 'loss of delicacy of feeling' inevitably consequent on the work made it totally unsuitable for the unmarried lady. If women wished to play any part in medicine, the journal suggested, they should take on the more 'legitimate' task of training as midwives for work among the poor, where, oddly enough, the 'physical disqualifications' it had considered an insuperable obstacle to their undertaking the better paid work of the medical practitioner were apparently of no consequence.[35]

This change of attitude towards midwives since the *Lancet*'s attack on the Royal Maternity Charity in 1854 may have been occasioned by the publicity recently given to that Charity's very favourable results.[36] But it is more than likely that the new threat of 'Petticoat Physic'—a greater evil to the profession than Sairey Gamp—played a larger part in this conversion. For the *Lancet*, and the many medical men who shared its views, the only permanent place for woman in the medical field was not as an equal competing for the fees of better-off patients, but as a helpmeet in the subordinate role of the nurse, or performing the 'true womanly' duty of visiting the bedsides of the sick poor. Though the midwife still existed, she was not seen as a serious long-term challenge to the profession. Those who worked for hospitals and infirmaries or for the larger outdoor charities (which still, however, served only a tiny fraction of the population) were subordinate to the institution's medical staff, while the practice of midwives working on their own account was everywhere declining. But the medical woman was different. Once admitted, she would be a permanent feature of the scene; male self-esteem—and male pockets too, it was thought—would suffer more from her competition than from that of the midwife who, as society became more affluent, was confidently expected to disappear.[37]

By the autumn of 1865 it appeared that 'Petticoat Physic' might be nearer than its opponents had supposed. That September

Elizabeth Garrett, the twenty-nine-year-old daughter of a Norfolk merchant, had passed the examination of the Society of Apothecaries. Her success (she had passed with flying colours) had demonstrated that contrary to popular belief women were capable of qualifying for the Register. But the way for Elizabeth had been long and hard. Denied access to recognized medical schools, she had been forced to pay high fees for private tuition, and when she had first applied to take the Apothecaries' examination the Society had refused to examine her. However, since the 1815 Apothecaries Act spoke of 'persons', women could not be legally excluded from its examinations. But it was not until threatened by a law-suit by Newson Garrett, Elizabeth's father, that the Society finally gave in.[38]

Miss Garrett soon became a successful practitioner. Her services were sought both by the well-to-do, and by the poor, who flocked to her Marylebone Dispensary for Women and Children. But the Apothecaries, determined that no other woman should qualify by the same route, hastened to amend their regulations so that in future nobody who had studied privately might be admitted to their examinations. For the time being, at least, the woman who wanted an independent career in the medical field must obtain her medical education abroad or rest content with the increasingly circumscribed and worse-paid work of the midwife.

While the medical profession was digesting the news of Miss Garrett's admission to the Register, another development threatened the peace of mind of those who wanted to see women kept out of medicine. In October of the same year there appeared in *The Times* a report of a 'Ladies' Medical College', which had opened in London the previous autumn with a dozen or so 'lady pupils'.[39] The College had been founded by an organization formed three years previously, in 1862, under the title of the 'Female Medical Society', and was now established at No. 4, Fitzroy Square. Among the Society's committee members were George Morant, the author of the pro-midwife *Hints for Husbands*, and Job Caudwell, publisher of a number of such pamphlets attacking male practice in midwifery. The Society was also fortunate in gaining the support of Professor F. W. Newman, a leading social reformer active in the feminist and temperance movements, and later in the battle against the Contagious Diseases Acts.

As its name implied, the Society hoped ultimately to secure the admission of women to the medical profession.[40] Its immediate goal, however, was the rehabilitation of midwifery as an occupation for gentlewomen—a goal for which the opponents of male practice had vainly striven for over sixty years. Perhaps, at last, the outside help so desperately needed if the midwife was ever to be reinstated was at hand. Significantly, the issue had not so far been taken up by the leaders of the feminist movement, who, single-mindedly setting their sights on the 'higher' position of medical woman, judged it best to have nothing to do with midwives.[41]

The Society justified itself in a number of ways. Midwives, it pointed out, were 'in charge' of the lives and health of a large section of the population, yet they had so far been unable to obtain training of the standard now provided by the Society's College. Further, by turning out well-trained lady accoucheurs from the College, the Society planned to provide skilled female practitioners for 'ladies' wishing to be attended by one of their own sex, a development called for by 'grave social and domestic considerations'. At the same time, it would be opening up a wide field of honourable and lucrative employment to educated women who would otherwise have been forced to seek work as governesses and who could not have been induced to take up midwifery under pre-existing conditions.[42] Not surprisingly, the feminist *Victoria Magazine* hailed the foundation of the Society's College as marking 'a new era' in the history of the midwife.[43]

The moving spirit in the foundation and subsequent running of the College was a thirty-two-year-old medical man, Dr. James Edmunds, at whose house in Fitzroy Square the College had its premises. The son of an Independent minister in East London, Dr. Edmunds had been for several years in general practice there before moving to the West End as a consultant. He had also for some years been a district surgeon for the Royal Maternity Charity, and had achieved the distinction of performing one of the few completely successful Caesarean operations. Like many other leading workers for women's rights, Dr. Edmunds was an advocate of temperance reform, and was later involved in the foundation of the London Temperance Hospital and the British Medical Temperance Association. His career, like that of Professor Newman, also provides an interesting illustration of the important connection between these two movements.[44]

Dr. Edmunds' experience with the Royal Maternity Charity had impressed him with its low maternal death rate compared with London as a whole, where attendance by men predominated.[45] An early disciple of Semmelweis at a time when the latter's work on antisepsis in midwifery was still viewed with suspicion by many leading obstetricians, he was convinced that much unnecessary maternal mortality arose from infection carried by medical men from their medical and surgical cases, and from post-mortem examinations. It was to separate midwifery from medical practice, as well as to spare 'delicate-minded' women the 'ordeal' of male attendance, that he wished to see a large-scale restoration of mid-wifery to women.[46]

Substantial benefits, Dr. Edmunds argued, would follow both to the public and to the profession from such a change. Midwifery was a time-consuming occupation, which interfered with a medical man's other work, broke into his leisure and destroyed his rest. No sooner did the best general practitioners achieve a 'large and respectable' clientele, than they employed a less experienced deputy for midwifery work, or fixed their fees at a prohibitive rate. Yet contrary to popular belief women were quite as intelligent and courageous as men, and were fully as capable of midwifery practice. All ordinary cases should therefore be handed over to well-instructed midwives of good education who would call in 'well known obstetricians' where there was difficulty or danger. Appealing to medical men to remember their sisters as well as their brothers, Dr. Edmunds reminded them that the womenfolk of many medical families were put to desperate shifts on the death or disablement of the breadwinner and that midwifery could provide such women with the means to maintain themselves in independence.[47] But although supporting those women who wished to become fully qualified medical practitioners, Dr. Edmunds did not think that anyone—male or female—who undertook midwifery should attend medical or surgical cases.[48]

The first step, Edmunds urged, was to provide for the better training of midwives. The training obtainable in the lying-in hospitals, he complained, was very deficient, and certificates of proficiency were often signed by medical men who had never seen the candidate. Furthermore, it was an anomaly that in England midwives were not subject to State regulation, as they were on the Continent. However, once it had established proper means of instruction and gained sufficient public support, the Female Medical Society would bring forward proposals for a complete scheme of midwife regulation.[49]

The Society's founders knew that if they were to succeed in this ambitious plan their pupils had to be of unimpeachable character and of acceptable social status, and it was not for nothing that they had named their school the '*Ladies*' Medical College'. Moreover, these women had to be prepared to risk affronting the current conventions which forbade the study and practice of midwifery to gentlewomen. By the autumn of 1865, however, twenty such students were attending the College. A few were 'ladies of position' seeking information useful to them in country areas or foreign travel, but most were women from professional families who were seeking a livelihood, and some were midwives already in practice who had gladly availed themselves of this opportunity of systematizing and improving their knowledge.[50] In consideration of the straitened circumstances of many of the pupils the course was offered at the subsidized rate of ten guineas.[51]

But it was not enough for success to find 'superior' women willing to become midwives. If they were to attract better-off patients, the instruction they received had to be at least comparable to that available to men and cover not only midwifery but the diseases of women and children. The course offered by the College included two winter lecture sessions on these subjects, delivered by Dr. E. W. Murphy, formerly Professor of Obstetrics at University College. According to Dr. Edmunds, these lectures were exactly the same as those given by Dr. Murphy to his male students as part of the authorized curriculum at the University, and, moreover, the standard of the College's teaching was higher than that demanded by the Society of Apothecaries. Practical experience was to be obtained at a lying-in hospital or charity in the intervening summer.[52]

The College was greeted with encouraging reactions from certain sections of the lay press, and with enthusiasm from the opponents of 'man-midwifery' and the campaigners for women's rights. It soon acquired the support of Lord Shaftesbury, the well-known philanthropist and reformer, and Lord Houghton, a friend of Florence Nightingale and a trustee of the Nightingale Fund. Dr. Farr, of the Registrar-General's Office, welcomed the fact that educated women were again taking up 'this old business of their sex', not in opposition to men, but in co-operation with them. Whatever the opinion of the medical profession on women doctors, he was sure that it would be glad to see educated young midwives replace 'ignorant old women' throughout the country.[53] Finally, the Lancet, which had made a violent attack on Dr. Edmunds for his statement that doctors often carried puerperal infection from their medical cases (an attack for which, under threat of legal action, it later apologized), nevertheless agreed that there was 'ample room' for well-trained midwives 'at least amongst the poorer classes'.[54]

But the 'skilled Lady Midwives' of the Ladies' Medical College did not intend to restrict themselves to practice amongst the poor in order to oblige the Lancet. The majority of the College's students were single women or widows who intended to earn an adequate living at this occupation. Many had been governesses, or otherwise would have become such, and a number, like Miss Firth and Miss Hodges, Matron and Assistant Matron of the British Lying-in Hospital, were midwives or nurses already in practice. By June 1866 Dr. Edmunds was able to report that the 'lady-midwives' who had

completed the College's course were being 'greedily' welcomed by
the public. Moreover, they counted a considerable number of 'lady
patients' in their practice, and received fees comparable to those
taken by medical men.[55]

Since the College was proposing to turn out a new category of
well-trained midwives, it might have been expected that it would
have gained the approval of Florence Nightingale. But although
Miss Nightingale shared Dr. Edmunds' views on the need for highly
skilled women practitioners in childbirth, she was far from enthusiastic about the College's work. While conceding that its midwives
were the 'best taught' in the country, she still looked forward to
founding her own School of Midwifery. There she intended to train
her 'Physician-Accoucheuses', or 'real' midwives, who would be
capable of attendance on *all* cases, normal and abnormal. Ultimately
the School would be staffed by 'lady professors', an objective she
considered perfectly feasible in the light of the distinguished careers
of the many continental midwives who had won an uncontested
place in the field.[56]

However, the Ladies' Medical College could only turn out a few
well-trained women each year, and these would work in towns
among the better-off. The problem of the great number of totally
uninstructed midwives, many of whom, like Sairey Gamp, combined
midwifery with laying out the dead or depended on other menial
or rough work to gain a livelihood, would still remain. Moreover,
there was now evidence that the extent of midwife practice throughout the country was much larger than many medical men, basing
their observations on the more prosperous sections of society, had
hitherto supposed. Indeed, the majority of medical men who had
contributed most to discussion of the midwife question practised in
London, and particularly in the West End. Now an investigation
into the causes of infant mortality undertaken by members of the
London Obstetrical Society at the request of Dr. Farr led him to
conclude that midwives attended about 70% of all births in England
and Wales.[57] A third to a half of East End mothers were attended by
midwives, but the latter had been virtually driven out of practice in
the West End. In small towns with little manufacturing industry the
proportion was thought to be quite low, but in large towns and
villages to range from a third to as much as 90%. According to the
Obstetrical Society investigators, most of these women, as Harrison
had found earlier in the century, had received no special instruction,
and were grossly ignorant and incompetent. Even in London, where
a large proportion had received some training, they were said to be
in general incapable of managing abnormal cases.[58]

Late in 1870 the Obstetrical Society made certain proposals on how the high infant death-rate, then estimated at 160 per 1,000 live births, might be lowered. Among the measures it wished to see was the registration of still-births[59] and the prohibition of *all* unqualified midwifery practice, male or female, with the immediate establishment of an Examining Board to test the competence of midwives.[60] On this last point there was little prospect of action, either from the Government or from the Apothecaries' or Surgeons' corporations, which, by virtue of the word 'persons' in their regulations, had the power to examine women.[61]

Early in 1872 therefore, the Obstetrical Society decided to take the initiative. Accordingly it set up its own Examination Board with its own diploma, hoping that this interim measure would ultimately lead to legislation. The examination was to be held three times a year in London, and was open to women between twenty-one and thirty who could produce a certificate of good character and who had undergone a course of instruction approved by the Society. Candidates must also have personally attended, under satisfactory supervision, twenty-five labours—far more than the number required of medical students by many of the medical examining bodies. The diploma received by a successful candidate certified her as a 'skilled Midwife, competent to attend natural labours', thus making it clear that she was not expected to undertake anything which the Society considered fell within the medical preserve.[62]

Reaction to the Society's venture was mixed. The *Lancet* and the *British Medical Journal*, whose editor, Dr. Ernest Hart, was actively concerned in the campaign for infant life protection, warmly approved. The *Medical Times*, on the other hand, was deeply suspicious of any step which might raise the status of the midwife to the detriment, as it feared, of the ordinary medical practitioner. Though the Obstetrical Society had made clear its opposition to the Female Medical Society's move to raise a class of highly skilled midwives, the journal took the opportunity of delivering a broadside at the 'hopeless spinsters' and 'sterile matrons' whose disappointments it implied provided the driving force behind the Society's campaign. There was no general demand for midwives in England, the journal declared, and in the 'exceptional' case of the few 'very impoverished districts' where patients could not afford the doctor's fees, such women should work only under medical superintendence. Grudgingly it admitted that the Obstetrical Society was as good a body as any other to examine the few required.[63]

Other critics included some of the despised spinsters who hoped to make a living out of midwifery. Many of these women condemned the Society's diploma as useless, since it qualified its holder for attendance on natural labour only, whereas they sought access to a publicly recognized qualification which would put them on an equal footing in midwifery with the general practitioner. Miss Nightingale, who was still hoping to establish her own Midwifery College, shared this view of the Society's diploma, considering that no 'educated Midwife' would come forward to be examined for it.[64]

Shortly after the institution of the Society's examination early in 1872 the issue of registration had been raised in the General Medical Council by Dr. Acland, Regius Professor of Medicine at Oxford. Acland, who thereby hoped to find a solution to the 'medical women' controversy, had for some time advocated the award of diplomas qualifying women to practise in midwifery and the diseases of women and children, and to act as Nursing Superintendents. Though there was some disagreement in the Council over whether it should concern itself with such matters, it appointed a sub-committee under Dr. Acland to consider whether it had power to register women as midwives, nurses, and dispensers.

Later in the year the case for midwife registration was brought to public notice by the appearance of *English Midwives: Their History and Prospects*, by Dr. J. H. Aveling. A recent arrival in London, Dr. Aveling had started his professional life in general practice near Sheffield, subsequently founding the Sheffield Hospital for Women (later the Jessop Hospital) in 1865. Three years later he had come to London to specialize in obstetrics and had started the Chelsea Hospital for Women, to which he was Senior Physician. He was also an active member of the Obstetrical Society. Aveling's book was primarily a plea for legislation for the control of midwives. Comparing their current position unfavourably with that of two hundred years before, Aveling pointed out that midwives as a body were incapable of bettering themselves without help from the public and from their 'stronger brothers' of the medical profession. He was convinced that it could only be people's unawareness of the widespread evil resulting from the ignorance of midwives that was hindering society from taking action. Accordingly, he challenged the women's rights movement to co-operate with medical men in tackling this *genuine* 'woman's question', and in remedying this substantial 'woman's wrong'.[65]

The already besmirched image of the midwife had recently suffered further adverse publicity during the trial of the 'baby-farmer' Mrs. Waters, hanged in 1870 for the murder of one of the many children who had died in her care. Also figuring in the case was a Mrs. Hall, a midwife. Mrs. Hall had kept one of the private lying-in homes which, as in Moll Flanders' day, still abounded in London, providing a refuge where women who wished to conceal an illegitimate pregnancy could obtain abortions or give birth in secret.

The unwanted children of these women were then put out to nurse, many being placed with baby-farmers like Mrs. Waters, under whose regime of neglect, starvation and slow poisoning they soon died. The bodies of such children might be dropped in the street or, since any person present at the birth might legally certify a child as still-born, buried as such; indeed, sometimes as many as three or four children were so buried under one certificate.[66]

Following these revelations, a Select Committee of the House of Commons was appointed to enquire into the problem of children put out to nurse. At the Committee's hearings several medical witnesses proposed the registration of midwives as an essential part of any scheme of infant life protection. However, this question the Committee considered to be beyond its terms of reference, and the legislation which followed in 1872 provided only for the registration of women fostering children for reward.

Proposals for midwife registration *were* currently being put forward, however, though on very different lines from those suggested by Aveling and his Obstetrical Society colleagues. Recently the Female Medical Society had announced its intention of promoting a Bill to allow suitably qualified women to be admitted to the Medical Register as 'Licentiates in Midwifery', a step which would have given them equal status with medical practitioners. At the same time a group of London midwives, which included Ladies' Medical College pupils, had formed themselves into an 'Obstetrical Association of Midwives' to further this object. The Association was led by the militant ex-matron of the British Lying-in Hospital, Miss Maria Firth, whose own career had shown that she did not consider midwives should restrict themselves to attendance on natural labour.[67]

The Association's first move was to request the Royal College of Surgeons to set up a Licence in Midwifery for women. But although the College had the necessary powers, it refused. Miss Firth then appealed to the General Medical Council's committee under Dr. Acland, hoping that it would recommend the institution of such a Licence, equal in status to that available to men. She also proposed that midwives should be allowed to sign vaccination certificates and, should the current proposals for still-birth registration become law, to continue to sign certificates of still-birth.

The Obstetrical Society also sent in its (very different) proposals to Dr. Acland. These were designed to prohibit practice not only by unqualified women, but also by unqualified men, and to place all persons allowed to practise as midwives in a position clearly subordinate to the medical profession. Registration machinery should be in the hands of the General Medical Council, which should be empowered to grant licences to persons passing the examination of the Society or any other approved examining body. These licences were to be renewed annually, on proof of good conduct; the midwife's status would thus be more comparable to that of the tradesman, like the cab-driver, stall-holder, or publican (for whom this type of control was traditionally used) rather than that of the professional, like the medical practitioner. By placing midwives under this stricter control, the Obstetrical Society hoped to suppress practice by persons likely to engage in the criminal activities—ranging from abortion to murder—described by witnesses to the Select Committee on Infant Life Protection.

Under the Obstetrical Society's scheme the G.M.C. would also have had the power to strike off women who attended abnormal cases without sending for medical assistance, thus reinforcing the superior position of the medical profession in midwifery. As Aveling was at pains to point out in the *British Medical Journal*, the Society's object was to improve the standard of midwives throughout the whole country. It would be impossible, even if the Society had desired it, to find in any numbers women capable of being trained to deal with abnormal as well as normal cases and at the same time willing to live in small villages and take the low fees which were all the poor could afford. The most that could be expected of women to be trained as country midwives, therefore, was that they should be healthy, and competent in the 'three R's'.[68]

Aveling himself was strongly opposed to the development of the highly trained, high-status midwife advocated by the Female Medical Society. In his opinion the Society's College fell between the two stools of medical woman and midwife. Its teaching was not complete enough to produce a properly trained medical practitioner, yet it aimed too high to play an effective part in providing the country with the 11,500 trained midwives which in his estimate were needed to attend the poor in natural labour.[69] Certainly the College's educated lady pupils would not entertain the idea of eking out a living by charing at the Hall or washing at the Rectory. Instead they would stay in the town and compete with the general practitioner for the better-paying patients.[70]

The committee appointed by the G.M.C. to enquire into its powers to register women as midwives, nurses, and dispensers, reported in April 1873. To the great disappointment of its Chairman, Dr. Acland, the Council proved to have no such powers. However, as other members pointed out, the registration of women dispensers was already catered for under the Pharmacy Act of 1868. (Indeed, several women were already on the Pharmaceutical Society's Register.[71]) Neither did members see any need to concern themselves about nurses; like Florence Nightingale, they considered that the improvement in the training and status of these workers would progress satisfactorily without registration.

There was more support for the registration of midwives, but it was the Obstetrical Society's view of the registered midwife, rather than that of Maria Firth's Midwives' Association, which prevailed. Professor Christison, though a bitter and unrelenting enemy of the women medical students who had recently attempted to qualify at Edinburgh, nevertheless looked forward with approval to midwife regulation. The provision of competent midwives, he declared, would present medical men with a 'golden opportunity' of ridding themselves of the onerous burden of poorly paid rural midwifery. But Dr. Acland's wish that the G.M.C. should itself undertake this responsibility was generally opposed as beneath the Council's dignity, or beyond its proper province.[72] Although his committee was reappointed, it did not report again, and the matter seems to have been dropped by common consent.

In the meantime the Obstetrical Society and the British Medical Association were seeking the support of the Government for the Society's own scheme. James Stansfeld, the President of the Local Government Board (now the department responsible for the Poor Law) had already expressed the view that registration of trained midwives would be of great service to his department,[73] and the campaigners accordingly appealed to him. But Stansfeld was a prominent member of the women's rights movement, and refused to consider a scheme which would have imposed such strict limitations on *all* midwives, no matter what their qualifications. He proposed instead that any registration measure should recognize two classes of midwife; a lower, subordinate one for the less qualified, and a superior one for the well-educated, highly skilled woman.[74] Worse still from the Society's point of view, he received with favour a deputation from Maria Firth's Midwives' Association, which was seeking just such an arrangement.

The Association had been thoroughly alarmed by the trend of events, and in a strongly worded *Address . . . to all Women Practising Midwifery*, it warned midwives of the danger they were in. Ever since medical men had discovered the advantages of 'Trades Unionism' and banded together in Societies and Colleges, said the *Address*, women practitioners had received less than justice. Now the Obstetrical Society's proposals for annual licensing of midwives aimed to weaken their position still further in the hope that shortly this 'necessary evil' would finally disappear. Were midwives so commonly guilty of immorality that they had to have tickets-of-leave like convicts? If such supervision *were* necessary, it should apply also to male practitioners, who were responsible for *more* maternal mortality than women, but who covered up each other's errors under the cloak of professional etiquette.[75]

Early in 1874 Dr. Aveling made an effort to gain more general support for the Obstetrical Society's scheme by reading a paper on the subject to the influential Social Science Association. Attacking the Female Medical Society's proposals, he warned the meeting that the more 'exalted' a midwife's position became, the more she would seek a better-paying class of patients; one he knew had put 'Accoucheuse' on her door-plate to discourage poor women from applying. Yet it was not this 'pseudo fine lady midwife' that the country really needed, but the woman who would be content to serve the poor—'the working, common-sense woman', who understood her business, and would wash, and mend, and cook and scrub as well, if necessary. However, she must be no more than a 'midwifery assistant', attending on natural labour only. There could be no intermediate class between this grade and the fully qualified medical woman, since full obstetric knowledge could not be obtained without a complete medical training. A midwife had therefore no more right to rank with the medical practitioner than a Bible reader with a Bishop.[76]

This view of the midwife was strongly challenged from the floor by Miss Firth, who resisted the notion that midwives should be prepared to do housework, and rest content with the 'paltry' fees of the poor. After this confrontation, however, no further mention of Miss Firth, or her Association, is to be found. Possibly her disappearance from the scene was linked with the closure of the Female Medical Society's College, which occurred about the same time. In the winter of 1872–3, the Society, which had the support of prominent figures like Shaftesbury, Archbishop Manning, the Earl of Dufferin (Viceroy of India), the Duke of Argyll and the wife of the Prime Minister, Mrs. Gladstone, had appealed for funds to extend the scope of its College, now operating in Great Portland Street under the title of 'Obstetrical College for Women'. The appeal had been careful to state that the expanded College could form a section of a full Medical College for women, should the foundation of such an institution become feasible. It may be that with this other proposal in the air, sufficient support for the Society's appeal was not forthcoming, and that its backers decided to join forces with the movement for the London School of Medicine for Women founded by Sophia Jex-Blake the following year. Whatever the reason, from mid-1873 the Society and its College drop completely from view. Dr. Edmunds, who had played such an important part in the foundation and running of the original College, had no connection with the new institution.

Thus, after a brief life of ten years, the Female Medical Society disappeared. But although it had failed in its object of providing the country with a continuing supply of highly trained midwives, and of securing their State registration, it had done an enormous amount for the rehabilitation of midwifery as an occupation for women. First, it had shown a generation brought up on Dickens' 'Sairey Gamp', that it was possible for educated gentlewomen to take up the work without losing their respectability, and had thus reopened a desperately needed avenue for their employment. Second, as even its opponent, Dr. Aveling, admitted, it had produced some 'excellent midwives',[77] and, as Dr. Edmunds was later able to report, many did 'valuable work' in various parts of the world.[78]

Furthermore, although the establishment of the new School of Medicine for Women meant that the pioneering work of the Female Medical Society was soon forgotten, the Society had helped to pave the way for the entry of women into the medical profession. Three of the women associated with the College went on to study medicine. One, Mrs. Isabel Thorne, became Secretary of the Women's Medical School, and another, Alice Vickery, became a well-known medical practitioner and a pioneer in the emergent birth-control movement.

But the disappearance of the Female Medical Society's College meant the end of higher training for a superior order of midwives, and consequently of any possibility that future legislation would confer official recognition on such a class. It was the refusal of Edinburgh University to allow Sophia Jex-Blake and her fellow students to continue their medical studies which had made her Medical School for Women necessary. But even if her School had not materialized, it is likely that the final result for the Female Medical Society's College would have been the same. Most influential obstetricians were against the Society's plans. They knew that any large-scale development of midwifery teaching in separate Colleges would put off still further the day when their specialty would be officially recognized as part of medicine, a step they considered essential for its continued development and for the improvement of their own status within the profession. It was also significant that Drs. Blackwell and Garrett Anderson, and many of the medical men who supported the move for a full medical college for women, were completely opposed to an institution aiming to turn out only partially qualified practitioners.[79]

Thus the hopes entertained by the Ladies' Medical College (and also by Florence Nightingale) that England would produce midwives who would achieve the scientific distinction of the great Continental midwives of the past were inevitably doomed. From now on women seeking a recognized qualification for the practice of midwifery on the same footing as medical men had to continue with the struggle to gain admission to the Medical Register as fully qualified practitioners. Even in France the rise of a new Lachapelle or Boivin was extremely unlikely; there too, midwives were gradually being brought under the authority of the medical profession, and opportunities for their instruction were becoming more limited.[80] In Germany, where the celebrated midwife Charlotte von Siebold had died full of honour a few years before,[81] midwives were more and more restricted to routine cases, and practice amongst the better-off was increasingly passing to men.[82]

It must not be supposed, however, that those medical men who had argued that women should only undertake the full practice of midwifery as qualified medical women would necessarily welcome these when they came. Certainly the Obstetrical Society did not. When in 1874 Dr. Elizabeth Garrett Anderson, who now had a considerable reputation, applied for membership of the Society, she was refused on the grounds of her sex. The Society, as the *Scotsman* newspaper pointed out, had thus formally declared its adherence to the 'most advanced principles of medical Trades Unionism' by deciding that no woman should take part in its discussions on the treatment of sufferings which women alone had to endure.[83]

The medical woman movement had derived a great deal of its support from those who believed that women were the most appropriate attendants in childbirth and in the diseases of women and children. But since the foundation of the London School had brought the admission of women to the Register one step nearer, it had become imperative for their opponents to proclaim the opposite view. 'Paradoxical' though it might appear, urged the *Lancet*, these were the very departments of medicine for which 'weak and tender women' were 'morally, psychologically and physically' the least well fitted. The thought of a medical woman getting out of bed on a cold winter's night, 'perhaps at a catamenial period', to walk or drive along a dreary country road to attend a midwifery case—whatever might be expected of the lowly midwife earning her tiny fee in the comfortless dwellings of the poor—was 'repugnant to a properly constituted mind'.[84] Furthermore, although it was unthinkable that men should be attended by women doctors—despite the sex of nurses—it was nonsense to suggest that a woman's modesty 'suffered' if she had to consult a man.[85] Yet had they been known, the private feelings of many of these women—like Queen Victoria's on 'those nasty doctors'—might well have supported a contrary opinion.[86]

But there was still a loop-hole through which the Edinburgh students might gain admission to the Medical Register. This was the examination for the Midwifery Licence of the Royal College of Surgeons. Under the terms of the Medical Act, the holder of the Licence was entitled to registration as a medical practitioner, and late in 1875 Sophia Jex-Blake and two of her Edinburgh colleagues applied to be examined for it. Since they had satisfied all its relevant requirements on training, the College could not legally refuse to admit them to its examination. But its midwifery examiners—all leading members of the Obstetrical Society—refused to conduct the examination, and resigned from the Examination Board. This action had the full support of the Obstetrical Society, which defended it on the grounds that obstetrics was an 'integral part' of medicine, and that it would be 'injurious' to the public if partially qualified persons were to gain access to the Register.[87]

Since for some years now the College had not admitted any candidate to its Midwifery Licence examination who did not already hold a qualification in either medicine or surgery, the Obstetrical Society's argument had some force. But to staunch Free Traders like the *Scotsman*, the Society's stand was merely another manifestation of the 'medical Trades Unionism' the paper had condemned on the occasion of Dr. Garrett Anderson's exclusion from the Society in 1874. Here was a Society of *men*, taking pride in preventing three *women* from gaining a qualification which was legally open to them, in a field highly appropriate to their sex, and in which they were exceptionally well instructed. To make matters worse, the reason given for the examiners' refusal was the candidates' lack of *other* medical qualifications for which the all-male medical examining bodies would not allow them to enter.[88]

Despite these reverses, however, the women's battle was nearly won, and within three years the citadel of male monopoly had fallen. The London School of Medicine for Women had gained access to the necessary clinical instructions at the Royal Free Hospital, and women might now qualify through the Irish College of Physicians, the Queen's University, Belfast, and the University of London, where the degree qualified the holder in all three branches of medicine. Gradually other medical examining bodies followed suit, and, though it was to be many years before all barriers were removed, the question of women's entry to medicine was in fact settled, leaving the way open for midwife registration to be debated as a separate issue. It was clear, however, that if midwives were to be registered, it would be as women qualified for attendance on natural labour only, at a level lower than the medical profession.

But there had been other significant developments for the future of the midwife. Before this period, the few spinsters entering this occupation were probably daughters of midwives already in practice.[89] Now, however, not only were gentlewomen again taking up this occupation, but a large proportion of these, like those entering nursing, were unmarried.[90] Some took up the work partly from religious and philanthropic motives, but many sought a livelihood. Since single women would on the whole have fewer family ties than married women, and would generally be younger, they could more easily seek training, and with a better educational background than most existing midwives, profit more from it.

However, there was another and more important consequence of this new influx. As Miss Firth's Association had shown, educated women could readily unite to protect their interests—something which for two-and-a-half centuries midwives had been unable to do. Now, at last, there was again a class of highly educated and vocal midwives capable of forming a pressure group for the advancement of their calling. It was the leaders of this new class—in contrast to midwives' spokeswomen of earlier times, mostly single women—who in the next three decades were to play a vital part in the ultimately successful battle for the reinstatement of midwifery as a respectable occupation for Englishwomen.

CHAPTER FIVE

Midwives for the Poor

The admission of women to the medical profession represented a spectacular victory for the women's rights movement. But there had been other gains also. In the late 1870s the general employment prospects of the middle-class girl were much brighter than they had been twenty years before. Women now worked in the Post Office as counter clerks and telegraphists, and there were increasing opportunities for female clerks and book-keepers in commerce and in the Civil Service. Nursing, too, had become a respectable occupation, in which educated women could look forward to positions of responsibility and influence. Though on the political front attempts to gain the Parliamentary franchise had failed, the first women members had been elected to sit on the new School Boards and on Boards of Guardians.

While the object of the women's movement was to enlarge the range and scope of female employment, the danger was that current proposals for midwife registration might restrict it. The scheme which the Obstetrical Society hoped to persuade the Government to embody in a Midwives Bill would have placed midwives under the control of a rival class, restricting them to attendance on natural labour only, and prohibiting practice by all but registered women. Though a ban on unqualified practice had not been included in the Medical Act, a precedent did exist in the 1815 Apothecaries Act, still sporadically enforced. More recently, however, there had been the example of the 1868 Pharmacy Act (largely inspired by John Simon, Medical Officer to the Privy Council) which had amended the law relating to the registration of chemists and druggists, and had forbidden the dispensing of drugs by unqualified persons.

Over the past twenty years too, the State had become more ready to intervene on health grounds in the lives of the general public. Legislation for the regulation of hours and conditions of work in factories and workshops had been considerably extended, and—a novel interference with traditional British liberties—under the 1853

Act the vaccination of infants had been made compulsory, with penalties for parental non-compliance. A similar invasion of English liberties was to be found in the Contagious Diseases Acts (1864, 1866 and 1869) which required prostitutes in garrison towns and sea-ports to undergo medical examinations (and if infected, detention in hospital) and had established a special corps of non-uniformed police to administer them. In the field of sanitation, the Act of 1866 had granted great new powers to nuisance removal authorities, and, more important, a duty to enforce them. Six years later the founda-tion of the modern public health system was to be laid with the establishment throughout the country of sanitary districts, each with a Medical Officer of Health, and operating under the oversight of the new central department responsible for Poor Law and public health matters, the Local Government Board.

Of all this legislation, most pertinent to women's affairs were the Contagious Diseases Acts and the Acts regulating the hours and conditions of women's work, and it is not surprising that there were many among the women's movement who were bitterly opposed to these measures. Primarily concerned with the removal of limitations on women's work and liberties, the movement was in general opposed to any attempt to impose new restrictions on women, whether they were represented as being in the interests of women themselves, or of the wider public. It was this determination which provided much of the impetus for the ultimately successful campaign against the Contagious Diseases Acts, and for the movement's con-tinuing opposition to the labour legislation which, in the name of protecting women, reduced or removed altogether their chances of earning a living.[1]

It was because the women's movement was generally opposed to legislation which placed restrictions on women's work that the Obstetrical Society's midwife registration scheme had not received its support. This coolness was a sore point with the Obstetrical Society, unable to understand why those concerned with women's rights would not work for a scheme which in its view was clearly designed to benefit so many of their sex. In 1874 the Society's President, Dr. E. J. Tilt, in his annual address to the Society, expressed his bewilderment and exasperation. Why, he demanded, were these 'noisy women' clamouring for the right to vote, and for the right to walk the hospitals alongside men, while neglecting a *true* 'woman's question'? Why, instead of seeking to assume the 'burdens' of men, did they not use their 'newly acquired eloquence' to campaign on behalf of their poorer sisters for that 'first right of all women', the right to safe childbirth? This task, however, they left to men.[2]

One of the objects of the 'noisy women' had been to break the male monopoly in medicine and in better paid midwifery—hence their resistance to proposals to restrict midwives to a low level of competence, and, consequently, of remuneration. The Obstetrical Society, on the other hand, had made plain its intention of securing the removal of the 'privileges' (of attending abnormal labours and using instruments) to which in their view midwives, however skilled, had no 'rights'.[3] For this reason the Society's registration scheme, together with succeeding ones based on the same principle, was to meet with persistent opposition from within the women's movement.

Though officially approved by the British Medical Association the Society's scheme had its medical critics, two of whom, Drs. G. T. Gream and A. B. Steele, were members of the Society, and consultants of high standing. In their view, the scheme was part of a general movement for the 're-introduction' of women into midwifery, of which the attempt to enrol Elizabeth Garrett Anderson into the Society was another. Midwives with any kind of certificate would impose on the credulous, usurping the position of the medical practitioner; it was thus 'humiliation' for the profession to see medical men of position testifying to the efficiency of women as medical advisers—which was what the registered midwife would turn out to be. It was not enough to say that midwives should be given legal recognition because they were widely employed; so, too, were bone-setters and prescribing druggists—should these be registered as well? Lastly, the least creditable part of the scheme was that these 'pseudo-obstetricians' who would not be considered good enough to attend the rich were being put forward as adequate for practice among the poor.[4]

Other medical opponents feared that registration would harm both the profession, which would lose practice to the registered midwife, and the public, which would suffer from her inferior services. Expounding the popular middle-class faith that by the practice of self-denial and thrift working-men could provide for all but exceptional misfortune, they considered that it was only 'reckless improvidence' which prevented them from making provision for paying the doctor through a provident club or dispensary. Midwives —and midwife registration—were therefore unnecessary.[5]

Others again doubted if registration would achieve what was expected of it, or even that the abuses it was designed to remedy were as extensive as its advocates claimed. The Medical Act, it was argued, had failed to drive out men who were far more dangerous than midwives. Many of these women did their work for nothing, or merely a glass of gin, and never did any harm. Though a large proportion could not read or write, they were to be preferred to literate women, who might read the letters of the ladies they attended, or make out false death certificates. In addition there was the question of the supply of these trained and registered midwives. What inducement was to be offered to persuade country women to pay for training, go up to London, and pass an examination, if all they could look forward to on their return was a few 5s. fees? In Ireland the provision of trained midwives was the responsibility of the County Authorities, which could each year send up women to the Rotunda for training, paid for out of the rates. In England no such system existed, and until this and similar organizational problems were resolved the plan would remain premature. It would in any case be 'cruel' to stop the 'friendly office' of neighbours, and the matter of midwife training could be safely left as it was, to be obtained through lying-in institutions and private practitioners on a voluntary basis.[6]

Dr. Aveling, who as Examiner of Midwives for the Obstetrical Society had been much involved in planning its scheme, came forward to defend it. Aveling welcomed the critics' interest, expressing his relief that no better arguments had been put forward against registration, and that its opponents had been so few. There was no basis for their alarm, however, and Messrs. Gream and Steele should realize that the word 'midwife' now had a different meaning from that of a generation ago. The Society was not proposing that the registered midwife should be regarded as competent to attend on all labours, normal or abnormal. Midwives were not to be regarded as equals and, therefore, as rivals, but merely as competent watchers of what was usually a natural process, and as useful assistants should emergencies occur. It would be a slur on the profession if it did not help to make those working 'in a parallel or lower groove' as capable and as serviceable as possible. Though Dr. Steele had quoted Dr. Tyler Smith's 1849 pronouncement that 'All midwives are a mistake', Tyler Smith himself had abandoned this 'optimist view' as his judgement had ripened and he had realized its impracticality. Aveling doubted if it was within the means of all poor women 'above the class of paupers' to pay the doctor's guinea. If a woman had a careful husband, it might be possible for her to save sixpence a week towards this, but in most cases this would never be done, even with the general institution of provident societies or savings banks.[7] Indeed, as subsequent surveys of urban poverty were to demonstrate, for a large proportion of the working-class it was a bitter and unremitting struggle to keep body and soul together, without putting by for the future.[8] For the agricultural labourer, also, who had a family to support, the guinea for midwifery was a very large sum to find out of a wage of 15s., or even less.[9]

Moreover, a large number of provident societies were run on unsound actuarial principles, and as a result were short-lived. Not all provided medical insurance, and of those that did, many gave no cover for midwifery attendance. Where benefit was paid, it appears often to have amounted to no more than ten shillings, or half the doctor's usual fee, and sometimes less.[10] In the case of provident dispensaries, subscribers might be faced with an extra charge of perhaps fifteen shillings for the attendance of the dispensary doctor.[11]

But even if most working-class women *were* able to provide for themselves in this way, it was unlikely that medical men would welcome all this exhausting and unremunerative work. Aveling himself related how his own experience of the 'miseries' of a large 'ten shilling' midwifery practice in a mining area had convinced him of this. Continuous attendance day and night on women of a 'humble' class, he thought, had an 'unmistakably deteriorating effect on the medical practitioner, mentally, morally, physically and pecuniarily'. Although midwifery was justly regarded as the 'key' to general practice, once a man was established he should hand over to the midwife all patients who could not pay remunerative fees. If those too poor to make provision for the doctor's guinea were nevertheless to be attended by a medical man, the only course would be to force them to apply to the Guardians for the services of the Poor Law doctor, which would 'pauperise' not only the patient, but the unemployed midwives as well.[12]

Such an arrangement would, in fact, have necessitated a major change of policy on the part of the Guardians, who as representatives of the ratepayers were generally reluctant to increase the burden on the rates. On the contrary, many Boards did not allow midwifery attendance by the Poor Law doctor, even in cases of great poverty, unless there were already four or five children in the family. Indeed, to many medical men the suggestion that more women should be attended under the Poor Law would have appeared a very unsatisfactory solution. Receipt of poor relief, even in the form of medical care in sickness, was widely believed to undermine an individual's will to lead an independent life, and to encourage idleness at the ratepayer's expense. The current industrial depression had led to a considerable rise in the number of paupers, and official Poor Law policy was to cut down all out-door relief to a minimum. Proposals were even made that medical relief, at least in towns, should be given only inside the workhouse.[13] It would thus have been impossible at this period to have secured an extension of Poor Law midwifery services, and Aveling and his colleagues were careful to argue that the implementation of their scheme would result in a *reduction* in the Poor Rate, as fewer families would be thrown on the parish through the death or disablement of the mother.[14]

But although the advocates of midwife regulation were agreed that the untrained, unsupervised midwife was responsible for much avoidable maternal mortality, there were no mortality figures relating to midwife practice as such. However, statistics did exist for the practice of midwives in out-door charities, who, as in the Royal Maternity Charity, worked under the oversight of their Medical Officers. Indeed, a number of charities showed a rate of less than half the 5 deaths per 1,000 births estimated by Dr. Farr of the Registrar-General's office for the nation on a whole. Similarly low rates were claimed both by individual midwives in private practice, and also by individual medical practitioners. Just as many midwives fell below this high standard, so too did many medical practitioners, as Dr. Farr, citing a case of fatal incompetence on the part of a medical man attending a well-to-do patient, was at pains to point out in his 1876 report to the Registrar-General.[15]

The highest mortality rates of all were without doubt in the larger lying-in hospitals, periodically swept by outbreaks of the deadly 'childbed' or 'puerperal' fever, which regularly closed wards and contributed to maternal death rates as high as 28 per 1,000.[16] As Dr. Farr commented in his report for 1867, lying-in hospitals had been founded for the relief of poor women; yet, as a result of congregating them under one roof, mortality among those delivered in hospital was far greater than among women delivered at home. To Farr, and to many others who studied the question, the logic of the situation seemed inescapable. Lying-in wards should be converted into small units receiving one or two patients each, or closed down in favour of a system of out-door practice—a quite feasible solution in view of the tiny percentage of deliveries taking place in hospital.[17] A forcible plea on these lines had been made to the Governors of the Rotunda by Dr. Evory Kennedy, an ex-Master of the Hospital, in 1867, and it was to promulgate this view that four years later Florence Nightingale published her *Notes on Lying-in Institutions*. In Birmingham this step was actually taken; the Lying-in Hospital was closed, and replaced by a system of out-door attendance by midwives on the pattern of the Royal Maternity Charity, a change amply justified by the results. If all mothers had received care of the standard provided by such charities, commented Dr. Farr in his report to the Registrar-General for 1876, maternal deaths for England and Wales would have fallen by 2,600 or 65%.

The hospital system had its champions, however, among whom figured the eminent Edinburgh obstetrician, James Matthews

Duncan. Duncan's *Mortality of Childbed* (1870) was written with the express object of defending the hospital system and discrediting the Royal Maternity and other similarly successful out-door charities. How, asked Duncan, could 'educated accoucheurs', who generally lost five times as many patients, believe in these charities' 'Munchausen successes'? Their records must be at fault, otherwise it would follow that poor women, delivered in filthy slum dwellings by 'imperfectly educated' midwives or medical students, were at less risk than well-to-do patients attended in salubrious conditions by experienced accoucheurs—clearly an 'absurd' conclusion. Even the official estimate of 5 maternal deaths per 1,000 births produced by the cautious Dr. Farr he dismissed as an impossibly low figure, postulating an irreducible minimum of at least 8 per 1,000.[18]

Duncan's views did not go unchallenged, however. Dr. Braxton-Hicks, Physician-Accoucheur at Guy's Hospital, who based his opinion on the results of the hospital's out-door practice (2·5 maternal deaths per 1,000 deliveries in 1869) thought Duncan's estimate 'overrated'.[19] Hicks' view was shared by Dr. George Rigden, a Canterbury practitioner, and in Farr's words 'a very exact, methodical recording man', who concluded from over 4,000 consecutive cases which he had attended over thirty years that in 'good ordinary private practice' not more than 1 in 400 should die.[20] As Miss Nightingale pointed out in her *Lying-in Institutions*, far from throwing doubt on Dr. Farr's estimates, Duncan had created a 'very painful impression' of quite another kind about the practice of the 'educated accoucheurs' quoted in his book.[21] Returning to this question in a letter to Dr. Farr, Miss Nightingale went further, arguing that Duncan's figures might well provide evidence for the commonly held (and, as shown in the first chapter, long-standing) belief that it was among the rich that maternal mortality was highest.[22]

Though puerperal fever was the chief single cause of maternal mortality its aetiology remained the subject of controversy. Though admitting that it could be transmitted in some way from one patient to another, some obstetricians believed it could arise 'spontaneously' from the 'combustible' nature of parturient women. Some considered it specific to lying-in women; others recognized its connection with erysipelas, scarlet fever, and other septic conditions.[23] Treatment also varied, but even at the hands of the most eminent practitioners, was likely to include copious and repeated draughts of wine and spirits, while cheaper, though no less noxious, folk remedies like turpentine were also prescribed.[24] Though the work of Semmelweis was known, it was still generally treated with scepticism, and it was not until the importance of Lister's work on antisepsis in surgery was recognized by more progressive obstetricians that the application of a rigorous antiseptic régime in the foremost lying-in hospitals greatly reduced deaths from the fever, and so put an end to proposals for the replacement of hospitals by outdoor charities. Such strict precautions were not generally adopted by individual midwives or medical men, however, and it was not until the middle of the next century that this ancient scourge was virtually eliminated.

In 1875 the controversy surrounding this subject was brought to the notice of the general public by the prosecution of two midwives on the novel charge of manslaughter by infection. One of the two, a Mrs. Ingram, had been ordered by the coroner conducting the inquest on a previous patient of hers who had died of the fever not to attend any more cases until given 'permission' by a medical man. However, the practitioner to whom she applied shortly afterwards had agreed that she might safely attend the second woman (an indication of the division in the profession about the possible contagiousness of the infection) and on hearing this the jury acquitted her. The second midwife, Elizabeth Marsden, who appeared a few months later at Salford Assizes, was not so lucky. A local surgeon had warned her to destroy her clothes and leave off practice for a month after attending a fatal case; she had, however, delivered two more women, both of whom had died of the fever. Mrs. Marsden, who had already been remanded in custody, was sentenced to prison for six months.

News of these prosecutions was received in medical circles with some anxiety, some practitioners fearing that they would constitute a precedent for the prosecution of medical men. One of these critics was Matthew Duncan, who pointed out that the 'so-called' crime of these 'poor defenceless women' was confessed to by 'ingenuous practitioners' in the medical press almost every week. In a frank admission which shocked some brother obstetricians, Duncan declared that he had never given up practice for a single day; busy practitioners could not afford to do so.[25]

In the meantime the Obstetrical Society had gained influential medical support for the principle of midwife registration. That same year, the General Medical Council had considered the question of the admission of women to medicine, and though distinctly unenthusiastic about this, had come out unequivocally for legislation to regulate women practising as midwives.[26] The Society's next step, therefore, was to seek the support of the Privy Council, as the department responsible for the oversight of professional regulation, for their registration scheme. Since 1873 when the scheme had first been drawn up the Society had made some alterations. In the new scheme the G.M.C., probably as a result of its members' lack of enthusiasm for involvement in midwife matters, was no longer to be saddled with the actual task of registration but was merely to supervise a network of *ad hoc* medical boards on whom the responsibility for the examination, registration and discipline of midwives in their area was to devolve. These boards were to consist of local medical men chosen by reference solely to their position and seniority, and were to include the 'two Senior Medical Officers of the Lying-in Hospital, Infirmary or dispensary' of the Assize town where the board was to sit, the 'Senior Medical Officer of Health', and the two 'Senior Practitioners' from the district.[27] The regulation of midwives was thus to be placed in the hands of the established medical men of the locality irrespective of their actual fitness for the task or their ability as potentially interested parties to do justice to the workers under their control.

Following the example of the Acts regulating apothecaries and chemists, the scheme proposed that 'bona fide' midwives already in practice should be admitted to the register, but that thereafter no woman who had not taken approved training and passed the required examination was to be allowed to practise. In addition, all practising midwives were to renew their licences annually, and these would be granted by the board on production of a certificate of good character signed by a local medical practitioner, Justice of the Peace, or minister of religion—a requirement clearly designed to place them on a level with the tradesman rather than the professional. The local Registrar of Births and Deaths would have the duty of reporting any complaints about midwives to the registration board. The board might then report the matter to the G.M.C., which would have the power of suspending or removing a midwife from the register.

In contrast with Continental schemes, under which the registration machinery was financed largely by Government, which might also provide free or subsidized instruction, grants for pupils' travelling and maintenance, and subsidies and equipment for midwives working in poor areas, the Obstetrical Society's boards were to have no funds beyond midwives' examination and registration fees. Since these must be kept low in consideration of the poverty-stricken condition of many of these women, the resultant sums might well prove inadequate to finance the working of the system. But although this problem could have been overcome by giving either central or local government a part in providing the registration machinery, from the Society's point of view this solution would have had the disadvantage that the regulation of midwife practice would no longer be solely in medical hands.

The Obstetrical Society submitted its scheme to the Lord

President of the Privy Council (1877), now the Tory Duke of Richmond, and the Duke requested the opinion of the G.M.C. Here, however, the scheme met with severe criticism from the G.M.C.'s Medical Acts Committee, chaired by that experienced public health administrator John Simon, formerly Medical Officer to the Privy Council and now Crown representative on the G.M.C. Despite the precedent for a ban on unqualified practice in the recent Pharmacy Act, the Committee's chief objection was to the proposal to ban the unregistered midwife. This proposal, the Committee pointed out, was contrary to the spirit of the Medical Act, which, while giving certain privileges to practitioners on the Register, did not render illegal the practice of unregistered persons. Since the Society's scheme concerned only women, such a prohibition would create the anomalous situation in which midwifery practice by the unregistered woman would be liable to statutory penalties, while the unqualified man would be free to practise under the protection of the Medical Act.[28]

Simon's Committee was also critical of the Society's 'very imperfect' arrangements for independent local registration boards. In its view the duty of registration should be laid on local government authorities. These could appoint medical boards to deal with medical aspects of the work, and already had public offices for the conduct of business and funds from which to defray those expenses which midwives' fees would probably not cover. The powers of local government in relation to the licensing of lunatic asylums and the prevention of food adulteration might well prove a suitable precedent. Nor, in the Committee's opinion, should the G.M.C. take on the burdensome and expensive duty of supervising local boards; in 'so simple a matter' County registers kept by 'proper' local authorities would be all that was necessary. After hearing the Committee's report, the G.M.C. decided not to commit itself on the method or scope of registration, merely returning to the Lord President a general statement in favour of the principle.[29]

The Obstetrical Society had thus not received all the support it had hoped for. Next year (1878), however, the Lord President brought forward a Government Bill to reform the medical registration system. The Bill proposed, *inter alia*, that in future all practitioners admitted to the Register must possess qualifications in both medicine *and* surgery (not, however, in midwifery). Though the questions raised by these proposals were difficult enough, and were further complicated by the controversy over women students, the Lord President had attempted in the same measure to provide for the regulation of midwives—and also for that of dentists, already the subject of a Private Member's Bill in the Commons.

In its own proposal for midwives' registration, the Obstetrical Society had sought to place the local machinery under strong central supervision by the G.M.C., hoping thus to ensure uniformity of procedure throughout the country. The Lord President, on the other hand, considered the midwife question far too difficult to be dealt with 'in a strict or stringent manner',[30] and his own proposals were accordingly framed on a permissive basis. The G.M.C. was to be permitted (but not required) to draw up and operate its own registration scheme, while the same power was also to be granted to the multitude of unco-ordinated local authorities having powers of government and rating.

The weak nature of the midwives clause was a great blow to the Obstetrical Society, which feared that the G.M.C. would not be anxious to act on its proposed powers. Predictably, when the matter came before the G.M.C., Simon was as opposed as ever to its involvement with midwives, holding that for a relatively immobile class of the 'same social level as housemaids, nurses, and the like', only local regulation was necessary. In the event, possibly as a result of representations from the Obstetrical Society to the G.M.C., Simon was overruled, some members arguing that if the G.M.C. did not frame a scheme, some other body would.[31] But the question of medical reform once more proved difficult to solve, and the Government's Bill was withdrawn. Although reintroduced the following year without the encumbrance of the midwives clause, it was no more successful, and it was not until 1886 that the matter of medical qualifications was finally settled.

In the meantime the anticipated failure of the Government's efforts on midwife registration had already led the Obstetrical Society's President, Dr. Charles West, to conclude that it would be better to detach 'this simple practical matter' from the wider and apparently more difficult question of medical reform. In West's view the midwife question did not 'in the slightest degree' involve the interests of the medical profession.[32] Indeed, the only opposition expressed to the Government's proposals on midwives had been the Society's criticism of their lack of force. There was, moreover, the encouraging example of the dentists. Provision for dentists' registration had been included in the Government Bill on lines similar to those proposed for midwives, but in the same year a Private Member's measure requiring the G.M.C. to undertake their registration had passed into law.[33]

This augured well for a separate measure dealing with midwives, and early in 1880 the Obstetrical Society leadership cherished hopes that a Midwives Bill might soon be before Parliament. But 1880 was an election year, and the Society's next President, Matthews

Duncan, was not so willing to see it engaged in 'political' work.[34]
From then on although the Society was to advise from time to time
on various proposals for midwife legislation, and individual members
like Dr. Aveling were to labour tirelessly in this cause, its main
contribution to the improvement of midwives was to lie in its
examination, the only independent one in Great Britain. The
Society's diploma was a qualification of a high enough status to
set standards for institutions training pupils, and to mark out its
holders from the general body of women in the work.

But very few women were actually seeking formal instruction.
Only a hundred or so midwife pupils were being trained annually
in the Lying-in Hospitals in the whole United Kingdom,[35] and very
few (almost all of them, despite Florence Nightingale's gloomy
forecast, educated gentlewomen) had availed themselves of the
Obstetrical Society's examination.[36] After 1880, when the Society
established provincial examination centres, the number of candidates
began to climb, reaching over 140 by the end of the decade. During
the same period, the number of midwives training in the London
Hospitals also increased, though they were still greatly outnumbered
by monthly nurses[37] and, in the case of Queen Charlotte's, also by
medical students. However, at the Liverpool Lying-in Hospital this
situation was reversed, with appreciably more midwives being
trained than either of the other two categories.

Since the demise of Maria Firth's Midwives' Association in 1874
there had been no women's organization working for the advancement and improvement of midwives. In 1880, however, another
midwives' society was founded. Its work was to be of far-reaching
significance for the future of the calling. Though like Maria Firth's
Association the new society aimed to raise the status of the midwife
by the recruitment of educated women and by State registration, its
philosophy differed in some important aspects from that of the earlier
organization, and it was for this reason that the new body (ultimately
to be the Royal College of Midwives) was eventually to achieve its
objectives.

The originator and first President of this new organization was
Miss Louisa Hubbard, the remarkably versatile daughter of a
prosperous Russian merchant. Miss Hubbard was not a midwife,
but on inheriting her father's riches had determined to devote her
life to the extension of employment opportunities for women. In
1859 she had helped to found the Society for the Employment of
Women, and was also to be instrumental in starting the Teachers'
Guild, the Women's Industrial Council, the National Union of
Women Workers, and many similar ventures.[38] In addition she
published and edited the monthly magazine *Work and Leisure* (up to

1879 the *Woman's Gazette*), and the *Englishwoman's Year Book*, both
devoted to the promotion of women's work and education.

Co-operating with Miss Hubbard were three midwives. These
were Mrs. Hornby-Evans and Miss E. J. Freeman, Matrons respectively of the City of London and British Lying-in Hospitals, and
Mrs. Zepherina Smith, wife of the Professor of Surgery at King's
College, London. Born Zepherina Veitch in 1836, Mrs. Smith was
a clergyman's daughter whose family was active in philanthropic
work. Before her marriage she had trained as a nurse and nursed the
wounded at the siege of Sedan. On her return to England Miss
Veitch had become interested in the question of midwife attendance
on poor childbearing women. Accordingly, she had trained as a
midwife at the British Lying-in Hospital, where she had gained the
Obstetrical Society's diploma in 1873. The contribution she was to
make to the improvement of midwife practice and the advancement
of the calling, was later to earn her the title of the 'Florence
Nightingale of midwives'.

In contrast to Miss Firth, the founders of the new Society realized
that if they were to achieve their object they must have the approval
of leading obstetricians. From the outset, therefore, the Society
declared its intention of working in harmony with the medical
profession. To this end its rules made it clear that the Society's
midwives were considered competent to deal with natural labour
only, and required them to send for medical assistance in all difficult
and dangerous cases. Miss Hubbard also consulted closely with Dr.
Aveling, receiving his blessing and encouragement for her plans.

The name of this new association was the 'Matrons' Aid or
Trained Midwives' Registration Society'. This double title was
indicative of the dilemma into which the prevailing prudery had
forced its lady founders. The first title, 'Matrons' Aid', gave the
Society the acceptable appearance of a philanthropic organization.
The inclusion of the word 'midwife', however, was a different matter,
and was the subject of 'long and anxious' discussions among the
founding members before the question was finally resolved. Indeed,
Miss Hubbard herself never overcame her sense of its impropriety.
'My dear, I wish there was another word for you,' she remarked on
one occasion to a midwife member who was visiting her home, 'it
would be so awkward if we used it just when the footman came in
to put on coals.'[39]

If the word itself was not respectable, it was clear that the problem
which it represented was also one which could not be freely and
openly discussed. A few months before, a writer on women's
occupations in the *Pall Mall Gazette* had been advised by her friends
not to mention midwifery; she had nevertheless braved herself not

only to write on the subject but also actually to use 'the old Bible word'.[40] The same year Louisa Hubbard's *Work and Leisure* considered that it had to justify a discussion of this subject to its female readers by reference to its bearing on women's work.[41]

The inducement held out by the Matrons' Aid Society and its supporters to persuade educated women to enter midwifery was primarily the prospect of a satisfactory living. The *Pall Mall Gazette* writer had deplored the fact that midwifery had fallen so much into the hands of men, but was confident that educated midwives would find a ready clientele among the wives of clerks, tradesmen and 'poor gentlemen'. This class, though aiming at the 'dignity' of a doctor and nurse, could only afford the inferior kind, and often paid dearly for their carelessness; they were likely, therefore, to welcome the educated and respectable midwife who would competently discharge the functions of both.

But clearly it was among the poor that the midwife would find the bulk of her work, and according to the Society £80 a year could 'easily' be earned in such practice.[42] Though fees for Poor Law and charity cases were low, being no more than 4s. to 6s. in the country and 5s. to 7s. in London,[43] this work was to be valued as a stepping-stone to private practice. Private cases, warned writers in *Work and Leisure* and the *Englishwoman's Review*, should never be taken by midwives 'of standing' at less than 10s., while 'tradespeople' could be expected to pay a guinea.[44] But guinea fees, as a practising member of the Society pointed out, were rare, and a midwife who earned £80 a year attending the poor would need to take on a very large number of cases, often working in squalid and comfortless conditions for days and nights on end. Her fees might have to be collected in instalments, and there were many bad debts.[45] Eighty pounds a year, however, was comparable with the pay of an assistant schoolmistress in the new Board schools, and was double that of the women clerks recently appointed in the Post Office.

Resident appointments in Hospitals or Poor Law infirmaries, at salaries of £25 to £30 a year all found (the remuneration of an upper servant in a private household), were also recommended. However, a writer in the *Englishwoman's Review*, who described these as 'comfortable' and 'not overworked', cannot have had much acquaintance with actual conditions. At this period hours for both nurses and midwives were excessively long, time off irregular and uncertain, and the diet often very monotonous. According to Louisa Hubbard's *Englishwoman's Year Book* for 1889 nurses were 'systematically ill-fed and over-worked'. In 1882 a nurse at Queen Charlotte's Hospital complained to the Committee of Management about the hours and the food. (It was not until 1895 that nurses were allowed pudding every day.) The nurse was told that her complaint had no foundation, since the hours and the diet had been approved by the Hospital's Medical Officers, who were themselves on the Committee.

But if the Matrons' Aid Society wished to attract educated women to midwifery, it was not enough to present them with the prospect o earning a satisfactory living. It was necessary to make their position respectable to them, and also to a public brought up on the image of the ignorant, drunken Sairey Gamp. The baby-farming scandals of the early 70s had shown midwives in a sinister light, and, as the part of Mme. Mourez in the Eliza Armstrong case was soon to demonstrate, 'Mother Midnight' still followed her ancient calling.[46]

For these reasons the Society had to be very careful in its selection of members. These were to be women over twenty-five years of age, of the 'highest character and competence', who held the certificate of the Obstetrical Society. They must also agree to follow a strict code of conduct. This required that members should abstain from alcohol in the course of duty, and not allow its use by patients except when prescribed for medicinal purposes—no mean task in face of the popular belief that strong drink was essential to a woman during her labour and lying-in. Members were also to refrain from discussing the details of their work with non-professionals, guarding their lives and conversation 'not only from evil, but from the appearance of it', and remembering always that their reputation, and that of the Association, would depend on their behaviour.[47]

All this was essential if the Society was to attract the strictly respectable middle-class lady. Like reformers in the nursing world who dignified the nurse's work into a 'high and holy' office, the Society's founders appealed directly to the strong evangelical religious sense which provided the driving force for so much contemporary philanthropic effort.[48] It was in this spirit that the *Pall Mall Gazette* article had described midwifery as a 'sphere of usefulness' which was not only 'right' and 'natural' for women, but also 'especially sacred' to them.

Among the Society's philanthropic objects were an improvement in the general standard of midwife practice and the safer childbirth which was expected to follow. In what appears to have been an answer to Dr. Tilt's complaint about the absence of feminine support for the Obstetrical Society's registration plans, the 'Matrons' Aid' Honorary Secretary, Mrs. Elinor Bedingfield, wrote to the *Lancet* about her organization's objectives. *Lancet* readers, she thought, would be interested to hear that some of the 'women of England' (the contemporary feminist phrase) had at last become aware of the dangers incurred by their 'poorer sisters' at the hands of untrained and incompetent midwives, and were in consequence seeking to promote midwife training and registration.[49]

But besides seeing their members as having a mission to save the lives and health of poor mothers, the Society's leaders hoped that they might also wield a salutory moral influence over the whole family. Accordingly, members were advised to exercise the 'greatest discretion and propriety' in their conduct and conversation, treating their patients with 'gentle firmness', and checking bad language and 'violent and immodest demeanour' whenever possible. They should also encourage mothers in the spirit of the Society's motto, 'Vita donum Dei', to regard their children's lives as a gift from God, for which they were responsible to Him.[50]

Clearly, such an attitude would mark out Matrons' Aid midwives from their humbler co-workers. Poor themselves, ordinary midwives were not so likely to be convinced of the value of a new arrival to the harassed and ill-fed mother of a large family, and were in consequence often less than conscientious in seeing that the child lived. As evidence to the Select Committee on Infant Life Protection had shown, some were quite willing to arrange its early demise, and even at a later period a midwife's 'churchyard luck' could be an important recommendation in the eyes of her clientele.[51]

Despite its small numbers the Matron's Aid Society had started well, enjoying the approval of medical campaigners for registration, and even of Florence Nightingale. But Miss Nightingale's carefully worded letter of congratulation to Miss Hubbard made it clear that her approval was conditional on the Society's working for an improvement of midwife training.[52] Her private view was that the Society would do little to raise the status of midwives if it set its sights no higher than the Obstetrical Society's diploma, with its requirement of only three months' training. 'Hopes without training,' was her acid comment in the margin of the Society's prospectus, 'are poor things'.[53]

Shortly after the Matrons' Aid Society's official inauguration in 1882, a fresh attempt was made to persuade the Government to take up the matter of midwife registration. This time the initiative came not from the Council of the Obstetrical Society, though the latter had co-operated fully in drawing up the proposed scheme, but from the Parliamentary Bills Committee of the British Medical Association, under the chairmanship of Dr. Ernest Hart. Their draft Bill broadly followed the Obstetrical Society's scheme of 1878, but there were some important differences. Annual licensing had been dropped, and the central supervision of local registration boards, which the G.M.C. had been so reluctant to undertake, was now to be the duty of a specially appointed Board. Though the G.M.C. itself was to be spared this work, the fact that it was to appoint the new Board meant that it would have considerable influence over its policy. Moreover—a change which reflected the greater involvement of the B.M.A.—a number of seats on both the central and local boards were to be reserved for men in general practice.

In disciplinary matters, midwives were to be treated more harshly than doctors and dentists. Like these, they might be removed from the register if convicted of a felony or misdemeanour, or for professional misconduct. However, they were also to be struck off if convicted twice of drunkenness. Evidently the drafters thought it necessary to specify this offence to make sure that it received the serious attention which they considered it deserved.[54] Unlike the Obstetrical Society's original scheme, the Bill did not propose to prohibit the practice of the unregistered midwife. Thus only women who *chose* to register would be subject to the restrictions imposed by the Bill, and the rest would be free to practise exactly as before.

In June 1882, the B.M.A. submitted its scheme to the Lord President of the Privy Council, now Lord Carlingford, and the latter, declaring himself to be in favour of its objects, passed it on to the G.M.C. for consideration. At its June session the G.M.C. received a B.M.A. deputation, which in putting the case for its proposals, maintained that it had the support of the whole profession.[55] The evidence for this statement was slight, however. The B.M.A. had circulated its local branches, which had signified their general approval. But the Association's membership included only half the medical men in practice and probably the more prosperous half at that. As the leadership was later to discover to its cost, it could not be safely concluded that the members' views were representative of general medical opinion.

Recommending their scheme to the G.M.C., the deputation argued that the work which it would impose on the Council would cause it only the minimum trouble and expense, since most of the burden would fall on the local boards and the cost would be met by midwives' fees. This view was challenged by the more realistic John Simon, who reminded fellow members of the 'mess' the G.M.C. had got into over the registration of dentists—the result of another privately drafted measure. There would be even more trouble, Simon warned, in 'sifting' the characters of midwives, a large number of whom had been described by the deputation as 'drunken and disorderly' and horrifyingly incompetent. This task, he considered, would be much better undertaken by local government authorities, and rather than discuss the clauses of an 'amateur' Bill, the G.M.C. should merely state its principles and leave the matter to the Government.[56]

But Simon was not chairman of the sub-committee on the Bill, as in 1877. This was now Professor John Marshall, Professor of Surgery at University College, London, who took a more positive view of the G.M.C.'s functions. In his opinion the Council had been created to protect the public in medical affairs, and far from being degraded by undertaking responsibility for midwife registration, it would thereby be discharging a 'high and most honourable duty'.[57] This view, rather than Simon's, won the day, and the sub-committee's report approving the general principles of the Bill was sent to the Lord President.

So much represented progress. The Bill was now backed by the G.M.C., the B.M.A., and the Obstetrical Society. No dissenting voice had been raised in the medical journals, the Lancet hoping that now the Bill was approved by the G.M.C. it might speedily pass through Parliament.[58] On the midwives' side, the Bill also had the general support of the Matrons' Aid Society which, although very small (it had only 26 members in 1885), was the only mid-wives' association in the country, and was busy collecting signatures for its petition in favour of legislation.

In fact, in its anxiety for registration, the Society had probably paid insufficient regard to the dangers which the B.M.A. Bill held for midwives—every bit as real as those threatened by Chamberlen's scheme of two hundred years before. It was left to a woman doctor, Sophia Jex-Blake, to act as the champion of midwives' rights. Writing to the Englishwoman's Review, Dr. Jex-Blake pointed out that under the Bill midwives were to be examined and governed exclusively by medical practitioners, 'a rival class'. No midwife, however highly qualified, might sit on the proposed Central Board, nor on the local boards which were to admit to, and strike off from, the registers. Yet these boards might include medical men who had never taken an examination in midwifery at all. Moreover, midwives were forbidden to attend abnormal labours, yet it was well known that many skilled women were more competent to do this than the ordinary general practitioner whose training in midwifery, if he had any at all, was generally very deficient. In short, the Bill was drafted with reference to the views of medical practitioners rather than to those of midwives, or to the public interest. Midwives included within their ranks a few 'highly educated ladies', but also a very large number of 'laborious workers' whose daily bread was at stake. Yet, as unenfranchised women, midwives were unlikely to secure representation of their interests in the House of Commons, as the medical profession had done. Parliament should therefore make sure that no injustice was done them.[59]

In fact, the Matrons' Aid Society did have reservations about some of the clauses in the B.M.A. Bill complained of by Dr. Jex-Blake, and made representations on the subject to the drafting committee. But the tiny Society was in no position to take a militant line. There was no support for its activities among the great body of midwives nor among the public at large; it was thus dependent entirely on the initiative and goodwill of the B.M.A. and the Obstetrical Society. Moreover, Matrons' Aid midwives were drawn from the upper middle classes, and some of their leaders had private means. These women did not depend on midwifery for a living, and could afford to look at the question from a philanthropic standpoint, as they saw it. Their medical acquaintance (Mrs. Smith, the President, was married to a Professor of Surgery and lived in Wimpole Street) consisted largely of established well-to-do doctors who, unlike many general practitioners, did not regard the midwife as a competitor.

The B.M.A. had understood that the Privy Council had adopted their draft Bill after the G.M.C.'s favourable report, and that it would shortly introduce it into Parliament. But no action was taken, and two and a half years later the Lord President told a further B.M.A. deputation that a 'shorter and less compulsory' measure would be more acceptable to the Government.[60] This renewed disappointment now convinced the Bill's promoters that there was no hope of Government co-operation, and that the only course was to introduce the Bill as a Private Member's measure.

The following year (1886) brought the long-awaited measure of medical reform. Among other things, the Act provided for the election by the profession of direct representatives to the G.M.C., as distinct from representatives of the corporations and universities, thus in part redressing a long-standing grievance felt by many of the rank and file ever since 1858. It also required that all practitioners admitted to the Register in future must possess a qualification in midwifery as well as in medicine and surgery, thus raising the status of the specialty by granting it legal recognition as part of medicine. However, it did not render illegal practice by unqualified persons in midwifery or any other branch of medicine.

With the question of medical reform out of the way, it might have been supposed that the medical campaigners for midwife registration would be quick to take up the matter once more. But the initiative was left to the Matrons' Aid Society, now operating unashamedly under the bolder title of 'Midwives' Institute', and soon to emerge as an effective pressure group for the improvement and registration of midwives. Though in its early years the Institute's existence had been precarious, its membership, which included trained nurses and some lay members, was now growing steadily, and by 1889 had reached 154. The Institute was also arranging for medical men to lecture to members, and providing much valued club and library facilities in its own premises at 15 Buckingham Street.

In the last few years the Institute had also been extremely fortunate in acquiring some outstandingly able and energetic new members. One of these was Miss Jane Wilson, already an active worker for the Workhouse Infirmary Nursing Association. This organization, founded a few years before to promote the employment of trained women as nurses in Workhouse Infirmaries, was also concerned in similar work relating to Poor Law midwives, many of whom were appointed to their posts with only monthly nurse experience. Another important recruit was Miss Rosalind Paget. After several years' work as a trained nurse in general and children's hospitals, Miss Paget had taken midwife training at the British Lying-in Hospital, gaining the Obstetrical Society's diploma in January 1885. However, her value to the Institute lay not only in her personal qualities, but also in her connections. She was niece to the influential merchant-philanthropist, William Rathbone, Liberal M.P. for North Caernarvonshire. Rathbone had done much to improve nursing services in his native Liverpool, and was a close friend of Florence Nightingale. At this time he was playing an important part in the establishment of the Jubilee Nursing Institute, an organization financed with money donated by Queen Victoria from the 'Women's Jubilee Gift', which had as its object the promotion of district nursing and midwifery services throughout the country.[61] The help and advice he was able to give the Midwives' Institute, both in and out of Parliament, was to prove invaluable.

In 1887 the Midwives' Institute had taken another important step forward. This was the publication, undertaken jointly with the Workhouse Nursing Infirmary Association, of a small monthly paper, *Nursing Notes*. Through this, Britain's first nursing journal, the Institute acquired a means of propagating its views on midwife registration. Current notions of propriety still restricted it in its efforts, however, and its editor and proprietor, Miss Emma Brierly, was later to recall with amusement how lay subscribers had it sent to them in closed envelopes, 'for fear that one of their household might see the word midwife, and look for more'.[62]

The next year, with the encouragement and advice of Dr. Aveling, the Institute set about the work of gaining public support for midwife registration. Aveling himself had lately given the matter much needed publicity by an address to the Hospitals Association, a recently founded organization of governors of voluntary hospitals. There Aveling had restated his view that the registered midwife should be of relatively humble social class, content to live among the poor mothers whom she served. She would attend the mother and baby at the birth and for several days afterwards, also doing the cooking and cleaning—in fact, combining the function of the midwife and the modern 'home help'. But although training in the provincial lying-in hospitals was generally cheaper,[63] in the London hospitals it cost over £20, which placed it beyond the means of the married countrywoman who might wish to undertake the work to supplement her income. For this reason pupils at the London Hospitals were better-off women, of a class, Aveling considered, 'not urgently required'. However, he was confident that if ways could be found of providing cheaper instruction, more suitable women would come forward for training.

Aveling's image of the registered midwife was the direct opposite of that fostered by the Midwives' Institute. Though agreeing that she must be limited to attendance on natural labour, the Institute was committed to raising her status, and to persuading educated women to take up the work. It was therefore just as critical of the suggestion that midwives should do their patients' house-work as Maria Firth had been fourteen years before. How, *Nursing Notes* demanded, could such midwives maintain the surgical cleanliness of the hands, now recognized as so important in midwifery? There were other dangers, too, inherent in a policy of encouraging women of low general education to train as midwives. To give women who were likely to be susceptible to financial inducements the technical knowledge of a midwifery training would be to expose them to 'temptations'—temptations which *Nursing Notes*, with true Victorian delicacy, did not define, but by which its readers well understood the procurement of abortion. There was no such danger with educated women, however, since by 'inheritance and habit' these possessed an instinct of professional morality which could not be expected from the inferior servant.[64]

The perennial problem of providing trained midwives for the country still remained. In the opinion of the Midwives' Institute, cheaper training alone would not solve this problem, which was primarily one of the remuneration to be expected. Moreover, since unqualified practice would still be legal, the trained midwife would be subject to competition from local women. The spinster midwife from London, who like Miss Alice Gregory, the daughter of the Dean of St. Paul's, might be given to middle-class moralizing,[65] or who might be above making the husband a cup of tea, could well be regarded as 'too grand and stuck-up' by many of her prospective clients. Thus the trained woman could only survive in the work if she were salaried or subsidized by a local charity, or had a private income.[66]

The Institute's ideal solution, which, however, it realized was an impossibility in England at the time, was a guaranteed basic salary for the trained midwife working in poor districts, and particularly in the country. In some Continental countries the public subsidization of midwives working in such areas was commonplace, and, indeed, a similar arrangement was already operating within the United Kingdom, as part of the Irish Poor Law dispensary system. Under this scheme the Irish Boards of Guardians employed a salaried dispensary doctor, and in some Unions, a salaried midwife also. Her pay, however, was low, averaging £16 4s. per annum, and she was evidently intended to supplement her earnings by private practice.[67] But the reputed over-generosity of the dispensary system, which did not impose such rigid income conditions for eligibility as did the English Poor Law Medical Service,[68] would not have accorded with the individualist philosophy of some of the Institute's more prominent supporters,[69] and was probably the reason why the Institute did not advocate the adoption of similar arrangements in England.

Cheaper training could have been provided in Poor Law Infirmaries, the larger of which had sufficient cases to allow of adequate practical instruction. Yet in the late eighties only three Infirmaries took midwife pupils.[70] Though the cost in these institutions was much less than the £30 to £50 charged by the prestigious London lying-in hospitals—being only £10 for three months, including board and lodging—this sum was well beyond the class of women whom Aveling desired to see trained to serve the poor. Again, since such women could already practise *without* the trouble and expense of training, often commanding the same fee as the certificated midwife, it was doubtful if they would consider it worthwhile to gain a formal qualification.

Family obligations which prevented many women from leaving home for training were an added complication. Such women might attempt the Obstetrical Society's examination having gained their instruction privately from medical men approved by the Society. However, even if they were fortunate enough to gain this instruction, there still remained the examination itself. One London midwife, a Mrs. Layton, who was an active member of the Women's Co-operative Guild, relates what an ordeal this could be for a working-class woman in the 1890s. The doctors for whom Mrs. Layton had worked as a maternity nurse had lent her midwifery books and encouraged her to enter the examination. Both written and oral parts, she recalls, were held late at night. For working-class women, unused to the art of composition, the two-hour written examination could be a daunting affair. A fortnight later came the oral, which in Mrs. Layton's case took place after 10 p.m., in 'a room full of doctors'. Confronted by this display of medical expertise and authority, Mrs. Layton was too nervous to do herself justice, and failed to gain the qualification on which she had set her heart. By this time, however, she was already practising on her own account, and when a few years later the Midwives Act became law she was admitted to the Roll as a 'bona fide' midwife.[71]

In the light of the difficulties facing the working-class woman seeking a qualification, it was clear that if there was to be any considerable growth in the numbers of trained women working in poor areas, particularly in the country, they would need to be subsidized from public or charitable sources. Philanthropic provision for financing the training and payment of midwives and nurses for such work was, of course, not new; however, with the establishment of local nursing associations, encouraged by the newly founded Jubilee Nursing Institute, it was soon to increase rapidly. A few years later local government itself was to play a part in training, with the institution of midwife scholarships by some of the new County Councils. But despite the continuing expansion of voluntary endeavour, the problem of providing trained midwives for rural areas was never completely solved until the Midwives Act of 1936 made the provision of an adequate midwife service mandatory on all local health authorities.

As it was, the numbers of women trained in the London lying-in hospitals as midwives for the 'Poor' remained very low compared with those trained as monthly nurses for the 'Rich'.[72] Moreover, of the middle-class women who *did* train as midwives, many took work as monthly nurses, for which a midwifery qualification was a useful recommendation. But even for the middle-class woman the expense of midwifery instruction was a great disincentive, since with shorter and cheaper training as a monthly nurse she could take up more comfortable and better-paid work among the wealthier classes.[73] For similar reasons she might also prefer to train for general nursing. As a probationer nurse she could pay for her instruction and keep by her work in the wards, something which applied in midwifery training only at the Jessop Hospital in Sheffield. In addition, as a nurse she had the advantage of belonging to what was now regarded as a respectable and even 'fashionable' occupation.

However, both Dr. Aveling and the Midwives' Institute remained confident that registration, by distinguishing the trained midwife from the ignorant untrained woman, would encourage more suitable recruits to come forward. Accordingly, on Aveling's advice, the Institute embarked on a campaign to gain parliamentary support for a Midwives Act. This was no small undertaking in an age in which matters relating to childbirth were generally considered improper for discussion in polite society, especially by single women, and in which all M.P.s were men. The first step, therefore, was to enlist the aid of women of position, and hope through them to gain the support of their relatives and friends in Parliament.

To this end the Institute organized a number of 'drawing-room meetings', at which the attendance of the new movement's more influential adherents was well publicized. These signs of independent activity on the part of midwives were not generally welcome, however, and the *British Medical Journal*, worried that midwives might be growing too ambitious, felt the need to give the Institute a warning. Medical men, it declared, looked forward to the provision of trained midwives who would 'relieve the hard-worked practitioner of drudgery as unprofitable as it is fatiguing'; however, the Institute should be aware that the profession would not tolerate any usurpation of medical functions.[74] With a new-found temerity, the Institute hit back. Its object, Miss Wilson tartly replied, was to 'alleviate the sufferings and minimise the dangers' of poor lying-in women, not to free medical men of 'irksome' labour in order to preserve their professional morale.[75]

Miss Wilson had also been encouraging the Institute to take a more independent line about proposals for registration, and had invited members to study the B.M.A.'s draft Bill of 1882 to see if it met the wants of midwives as well as those of the public. But despite the power over midwives which the Bill proposed to grant to the local registration boards, with their preponderance of general practitioners, members concluded that the Bill was 'on the whole satisfactory'. They did, however, decide to ask for representation of the Institute on the central supervisory board (not considered necessary by the Bill's medical authors) by a midwife, or, failing this, by a medical practitioner. There were far more educated women working as midwives, Miss Wilson pointed out, than six years earlier when the B.M.A. draft Bill had first been discussed.[76] Indeed, the Hospitals' Association's new nursing journal, the *Hospital Nursing Mirror*, had commented on the significant fact that at the Institute's drawing-room meetings there had been 'elegant ladies' proud to accept the 'good old English title of midwife'.[77]

But the Midwives' Institute was no longer the only group of women actively interested in midwife registration. Since 1887 the situation had been complicated by the arrival on the scene of a new organization. This was the British Nurses' Association, founded by a group of lady nurses pledged to fight for the advancement and improvement of nurses, and for their registration by the State. At its head was the militant Mrs. Bedford Fenwick, a doctor's daughter,

who at the age of twenty-four had been appointed Matron of
St. Bartholomew's Hospital, and who was now the wife of a Wimpole
Street physician active in medical politics. Medical men were
admitted as members of the Association, and the leadership was
divided between them and leading nurses under the presidency of
Mrs. Fenwick. Early in 1888 Mrs. Fenwick founded her own journal,
the *Nursing Record*, which she used as a vehicle for promulgating her
forceful views on nursing and allied subjects, and in which she un-
mercifully belaboured her critics and rivals. The Association grew
rapidly and by the early months of 1889 was claiming a membership
of over 3,000.

Mrs. Fenwick had set her sights high. She aimed not only at
registration, but also at transforming nursing into a profession solely
for 'ladies' with three years' training. In this she was opposed by
Florence Nightingale, who considered three years too much to
require of the average nurse, and whose opinion on the merits of
registration had not changed. Also opposed were other leading
figures in hospital management and nursing. In their view registration would lower the status of the best-trained nurses (and consequently of the leading training schools) while doing little or nothing
to raise general standards. Among these opponents was Henry
Burdett, Secretary of the Hospitals' Association, which had established its own register of trained nurses. Between Burdett and Mrs.
Fenwick, both uncompromising and opinionated persons, there
sprang up a bitter and lasting animosity.

On the subject of midwife registration it might have been expected
that Mrs. Fenwick would give the Midwives' Institute her unqualified support, since a Midwives Act would have proved a useful
precedent for the registration of nurses. But this would have meant
waiting, and Mrs. Fenwick did not wish to wait. On the contrary, she
hoped to use the more mature midwives' movement to help her gain
a short-cut to nurse registration. She therefore invited the Institute
to join forces with the Nurses' Association in seeking a Royal
Charter to empower it to register midwives as well as nurses.

Indeed, Mrs. Fenwick's project held attractions for educated
midwives, some of whom had several years' nurse training, and were
already members of the British Nurses' Association. It was not
surprising that such women should have preferred to be officially
associated with Mrs. Fenwick's lady nurses rather than, as proposed
under previous schemes for midwife registration, be lumped
together with the poor, uneducated and untrained women who
would have constituted the bulk of midwives on the register. It was
with these educated nurse-midwives in mind that Mrs. Fenwick
suggested the institution on the proposed B.N.A. register of an upper

grade of midwife, in order that such women might be distinguished from the rest.

Furthermore, by contrasting the size and influence of her Association with the Midwives' Institute's mere 150 members, and confidently prophesying its success in gaining legal sanction for its registration scheme, Mrs. Fenwick managed to give to her suggestion of joint action the appearance of a benevolent favour to a poor and successful relation. But the Institute was not to be seduced, and Mrs. Fenwick's overtures met with a rebuff. In a firm letter to the *Record* Miss Wilson pointed out that midwives, unlike nurses, were independent practitioners in their own right, with sole responsibility for their patients. Their registration was therefore a more urgent matter, and should be dealt with separately.[78]

Mrs. Fenwick had her answer ready. On the contrary, she urged, the registration of nurses would be more immediately useful to the public, since only the class affluent enough to employ a nurse would actually buy and consult a register. Poor mothers who employed midwives would continue to engage the local woman, whether registered or not, and the 'earnest workers' of the Midwives' Institute were merely 'dreaming the vainest of dreams' if they expected Parliament, which for the last half century had followed the principle of Free Trade in commerce, medicine, and religion, to ban the unregistered midwife's practice.[79]

Despite the refusal of the Midwives' Institute to join forces with the B.N.A., Mrs. Fenwick was still confident that the Association would succeed in gaining powers to register midwives as well as nurses. In order to gain support for these objects, a large meeting was held at the Mansion House in July of the following year, 1889. There, to Mrs. Fenwick's great satisfaction, two eminent obstetricians, Dr. Matthews Duncan and Sir William Priestley, M.P., ex-President of the Obstetrical Society, and a long-standing advocate of midwife registration, urged this additional task on the B.N.A. But Duncan's statement that a 'midwife' and a 'midwifery nurse' were, after all, the same thing infuriated the Midwives' Institute. This was further evidence of the widespread confusion which the Institute had recently been attempting to dispel as to the difference in role between the midwife, an independent practitioner, and the 'monthly' or 'midwifery' nurse, who only undertook nursing duties.

The Midwives' Institute itself included members who were keenly interested in nurse registration, but it was nonetheless not going to be lured by the B.N.A.'s apparently magnanimous offer into abandoning its own independent action for midwives. Dismissing the 'success' of the B.N.A. as merely 'meetings' and 'talk',[80] the Institute had rightly judged that midwives were nearer to registration than nurses. Legislation for nurses was still strongly opposed by Florence Nightingale and other powerful figures in the hospital world. On the other hand, there appeared to be no opposition to midwife registration, which had the support of the G.M.C., the B.M.A., and the Obstetrical Society. Even Miss Nightingale, who was to checkmate the B.N.A.'s efforts at every turn, herself agreed that the case of midwives was entirely different. Hence the Midwives' Institute wisely refused to be deflected from its purpose, while Dr. Aveling warned the B.N.A. that their attempt to achieve registration by 'laying their egg in the midwives' nest' was bound to fail.[81]

A few weeks after the Mansion House meeting, one of the M.P.s supporting registration, Mr. Fell Pease, approached the G.M.C. to see if it were willing to nominate a Midwives Registration Board. But this time that body reverted to its position of 1877, once more supporting John Simon in his view that registration should be undertaken by local authorities under the oversight of a Government department. However, it agreed to give advice on the rules to govern registration, but—to the great disgust of the British Medical Journal— refused to take any part in the detailed arrangements.[82] Evidently most G.M.C. members agreed with Simon that these were a matter for the new County Councils, the establishment of which had finally given the country a nation-wide system of general purpose authorities. However, it was indicative of the suspicion with which general practitioners viewed Medical Officers of Health that this suggestion was resisted by Dr. James Glover, the only general practitioner on the G.M.C. Glover feared that to make County Councils responsible for the local machinery would introduce 'political considerations' into registration, and give too much power to Medical Officers of Health.[83]

But Mr. Pease's proposition was not the only one concerning midwife registration to be laid before the G.M.C. The B.N.A. had also put forward for consideration its own scheme for the joint registration of midwives and nurses. Emphasizing the superiority of their proposals for the 'professional' control of the registered midwife (by the medical men and nurses running the B.N.A.) over any involving lay control (the County Councils suggested as possible local registration authorities), the B.N.A. sought the G.M.C.'s support for their proposals. But despite the advocacy of two of its members, the G.M.C. refused to consider nurses in the same context as midwives. Though accepting that nurse registration might be useful, it declined to express an opinion on the methods to be employed, or itself to take any action on the matter.

Although this was a set-back to her plans, Mrs. Fenwick continued supremely confident that the B.N.A. would shortly gain a Royal Charter giving official sanction to its proposed registration scheme. Piqued by the refusal of the Midwives' Institute to join forces with her Association, she lost no opportunity of twitting it with its small numbers, and its slow progress towards its goal compared with the apparently rapid success of the B.N.A. It was the B.N.A., she claimed, which had forced the urgency of the midwife question on the attention of the public, and the 'gentle reformers' of the Midwives' Institute had only been 'galvanised' into action by the Mansion House proposals that the B.N.A. itself should undertake the task.[84]

This was unfair to the Midwives' Institute, which had been mounting its own campaign for registration before the Mansion House proposals were made. Moreover, although small in numbers, the Institute had built for itself a position as spokesman for midwives' interests, a position it had recently consolidated by its incorporation. This had already had practical results. Earlier, when the first registration proposals had been produced by the Obstetrical Society and the B.M.A., it had not been thought necessary to consult midwives. Now the Institute's President had a seat on the committee set up to frame the Bill, and £1,000 had been raised to defray the considerable expenses of a Private Member's measure.

Finally, in contrast to the B.N.A., which had a large and dominant medical element in its membership, the Institute was a women's organization, run by women, and independent of the medical profession. While it had neither the means nor the prestige to impress the public by holding meetings in the Mansion House, this independence was ultimately to prove a greater asset to the midwives' cause. All in all, considering its small beginnings, the Institute had no reason to be ashamed of its achievements to date on the 'woman's question' of midwife registration.

CHAPTER SIX

Medical Men and Midwives Bills

The failure of Maria Firth's movement for the registration of the midwife on equal terms with the medical practitioner had made it inevitable that any successful campaign must have the co-operation —or at least, the acquiescence—of a substantial part of the medical profession, and in particular that of obstetricians. It followed, therefore, that any Bill which was to have a chance of passing into law would have to propose to register midwives at a lower level than doctors, and that in consequence it would encounter resistance among midwives themselves, as well as from the women's rights movement. This prospect did not alarm the registration party, however. Apart from the brief opposition of a few doctors to the Obstetrical Society's scheme in the early 1870s, there had been no publicly expressed medical objections to registration on these lines. Their proposals had the approval of the Obstetrical Society, whose membership included leading obstetricians and general practitioners throughout the country, and of the B.M.A., with its network of local branches, and, finally, of the General Medical Council itself. Confident, therefore, that they enjoyed the support of the whole profession, the registration party was convinced that once a Midwives Bill came before Parliament it would soon be law.

In this they could not have been more mistaken. Ever since apothecaries had raised themselves from being humble dispensers of medicines to being respected general medical practitioners, they had feared that in the same way a new class would gain a foothold within the profession and undermine them from below. Hence the obsession of the general practitioner throughout the nineteenth century with the possibility that an inferior order of less qualified practitioners, like the French 'officier de santé', or the Russian 'feldscher', would arise to undercut him and rob him of his practice. It was this continuing fear which had inspired the alarm with which many general practitioners had greeted the registration of chemists under the Pharmacy Acts of 1852 and 1868. In poorer areas chemists not only prescribed for the sick, but often visited them in their homes, and many also practised midwifery. State registration, would, it was objected, encourage the chemist to use his 'showy diploma' to deceive both himself and the public as to his knowledge and skill and lead him to poach still further on the preserve of the medical profession.[1] In the event, however, the registration of chemists outside the profession precluded them from gaining an official position within it, as the apothecaries had done. The general practitioner in poorer areas still continued to complain about 'competition' from chemists until the financial barrier between him and his patient was removed by the National Health Service in 1948. Yet this was not competition in any real sense; in fact the chemist relieved the medical man of much profitless labour, since many of those who sought his aid in medical matters could not in any case afford the doctor's fee. But to the less successful general practitioner matters did not appear in this light, and for the same reasons for which this section of the profession had objected to the Pharmacy Acts, they could be expected to oppose the registration of midwives. Ever since men had taken up midwifery on any scale there had been many, especially in the lower ranks of the profession, who had pursued the midwife with a jealous and unremitting enmity, seeking always to limit and harass her in her practice and looking forward to her ultimate disappearance. Despite extensive support for registration among established leaders of the profession, hostility among the rank and file was to be the most important single factor in preventing the arrival of a Midwives Act on the Statute Book before 1902.

Early in 1890 the first of many Midwives Bills was introduced into the House of Commons by Mr. Fell Pease. Officially promoted by the Midwives' Institute, the Bill was the result of discussions between them, their lay supporters, and the Council of the Obstetrical Society. It was thus an attempt to reconcile different, and sometimes conflicting, objectives. All parties agreed on the need to provide a better midwifery service for poor childbearing women. But the aim of the Midwives' Institute was also to improve the midwife's position, and to attract educated women to the work. On the other hand, most medical advocates of registration, whether they saw a permanent place for the midwife in routine attendance on the poor, or only expected her to survive until increasing affluence enabled everyone to afford the attendance of a medical practitioner, looked forward to legislation as a means of restricting her role and reducing her to a position subordinate to the medical profession. In fact, the Bill largely followed the draft drawn up by the B.M.A. in 1882, and included many of its impractical features. The machinery of registration was to be placed completely under medical control—a matter of paramount importance to its medical supporters. Some of the Bill's lay promoters had evidently taken the view that this machinery should be provided by the new County Councils, working under the supervision of the Local Government Board. However, it was the Obstetrical Society's proposal of local medical boards, independent of local government, and without any subvention from public funds, which had prevailed. The very real possibility that midwives' fees would not be sufficient to finance the registration machinery had been ignored by the Society in order to keep this machinery in medical hands. As in the 1882 draft, the boards were to include a number of general practitioners, and were now to be responsible not only for the examination and registration of midwives in the area but also for their suspension and erasure from the register. Aggrieved midwives were to have the right of appeal to the proposed central Midwives Board or to the Privy Council.

It was also the medical view that the maintenance of uniform standards required general supervision of the local boards by a central medical authority. The obvious body to undertake this was the G.M.C., already responsible for registering dentists. But the G.M.C. had recently reaffirmed its repeated refusal to accept any continuing responsibility for midwives, and the promoters were left with the task of proposing a new authority to carry out this work. Their proposed solution was a compromise, designed to be as cheap as possible, but in reality quite impractical. The registration board for London was to exercise supervision over the provincial boards and the G.M.C. was to be asked to frame the rules governing examination, registration, and discipline. In recognition of its supervisory duties, the London Board was to be much larger than the others, but like them was to consist solely of medical practitioners, who would serve for life—not an arrangement likely to promote efficiency. Members were to be the senior acting obstetricians of eleven named London Hospitals,[2] ex officio, and one representative each from the three medical corporations, the Obstetrical Society, the University of London, and the Midwives' Institute.

The granting of a seat on the Central Board to the Midwives' Institute was a great concession on the part of the medical men framing the Bill, and was the result of the Institute's patient insistence on this point. Mrs. Bedford Fenwick—always a champion of women's rights—was to argue in her Nursing Record that the Institute's representative should be a midwife rather than a medical man.[3] But the Institute, dependent as it was on medical support, was not yet secure enough to stand out for this. Moreover, the strength of its leaders' determination to improve the general standard of midwife practice among the poor made them willing to sacrifice midwives' interests to this philanthropic end.[4]

In any case, although the Central Midwives Board was established to supervise women workers who were themselves to serve only women patients, there was no precedent for putting a woman on such a statutory body. Indeed, it was still generally accepted that women's interests could properly be represented, and, indeed, *should* be represented, by men. Women were excluded from the management of hospitals—even of lying-in hospitals[5]—and their participation in government was limited to membership of a few School Boards and Boards of Guardians. Nor would the appointment of a woman have been universally popular even among the supporters of registration. One pro-registration medical member of the British Nurses' Association was later to refer to his experience of a 'mixed' committee as something he would not care to repeat; the presence of women on the Midwives Board, he warned, would strike terror into the hearts of their male colleagues.[6]

The Bill won a place in the Private Members' ballot for 21 May. Among the M.P.s backing it were Miss Paget's uncle, William Rathbone, and three prominent medical men, Dr. Farquharson, Sir Guyer Hunter, and Sir Walter Foster, who was also Vice-President of the B.M.A., the profession's direct representative on the G.M.C., and Chairman of the National Liberal Federation. The Bill thus appeared to have solid medical support. No opposition to midwife registration had been voiced in the medical press, and the *British Medical Journal* seemed justified in claiming that the profession was generally in favour.[7]

Though the time for debate on the Bill was short, it was soon clear that it would be strongly opposed. One opponent was a medical man, Dr. C. K. Tanner, M.P. for mid-Cork. Though disclaiming any personal hostility to the Bill, Dr. Tanner felt obliged to speak against it on account of representations he had received from medical men in various parts of the country who feared that the registered midwife would rob them of a large part of their practice. However, if the Bill could be suitably amended, he himself would be content to see it pass.

The Bill was also opposed by two lay members, J. T. Brunner and Charles Bradlaugh, freethinker M.P. for Northampton. Both deprecated the increasing tendency to legislate for the regulation of people's lives, and while conceding that the Bill was intended for the public good, pointed out that it discriminated against women. Midwives wishing to register were to be required to produce a certificate of good character, yet no such demand was made of medical men registering under the Medical Acts. Technical competence should be the only test for admission to the register, Bradlaugh maintained. He was still speaking at 5.30 and the Bill was talked out.[8]

However, Government itself was now showing interest in the subject. Dissatisfied with the form of the Bill, the Lord President (the Conservative Viscount Cranbrook), had arranged for it to be referred to a Select Committee, in the meantime drafting a Government measure. It was the Privy Council's view that examination and registration should be in the hands of County Councils, since these were existing local bodies with public offices and the power to raise any necessary funds. However, the department charged with the oversight of local government, the Local Government Board, had disclaimed any interest in the Bill, contenting itself with pointing out to the Privy Council that County Councils might not wish to undertake these 'novel duties'.[9]

These proposals did not please the B.M.A. which, like the Obstetrical Society, took the view that the registration machinery should be entirely in medical hands. However, when faced with the Privy Council's opposition, they conceded the point on condition that the rules governing examinations and discipline were laid down centrally by the G.M.C. Although they would have liked the addition of a clause explicitly limiting the midwife to attendance on natural labour, they accepted the Privy Council's opinion that this complicated matter would be better dealt with in the rules to be made under the Act. Agreement had thus been reached between the promoters, the B.M.A., and the Government, and the Bill was duly amended by the Select Committee to take account of the Privy Council's views.

But it was too late for the Bill to be debated again that session. Moreover, since its introduction to the House in May, it had become clear that the B.M.A. view on registration was not shared by all the profession. Outright opposition—not only to the Bill but also to the principle of registration itself—had come from various sources. One was the *Provincial Medical Journal*, a monthly catering for the provincial general practitioner, in which several correspondents had expressed their hostility. The most vocal of these was a Liverpool man in general practice, Dr. Robert Rentoul, who had set himself up as the champion of the less affluent medical practitioner. Rentoul was already an active participant in the campaign currently being waged by a group of general practitioners against the 'abuse' of free dispensaries and hospital out-patient departments by persons they considered well able to afford the general practitioner's fee. With the same polemical zeal which he had brought to these other activities, Dr. Rentoul now began a relentless war against the

Midwives Bill in the columns of the medical journals,[10] in the B.M.A. itself, and in any other arena in which he could gain a hearing.

Ironically, in view of the marked anti-feminism of some medical advocates of registration, and the past reaction of the women's rights movement to their proposals, Rentoul attacked the registration campaign as a deep-laid feminist plot to drive men out of midwifery. The Midwives Bill, he protested, was just one more stage along the road leading to the extinction of general practice. Dentistry had already been 'given away' by the profession (a reference to the separate registration of dentists in 1878), and pharmacy was no longer a respectable part of medicine. Now the registered midwife would rob the general practitioner of a large part of his income, and thus speedily accomplish his complete destruction.

Obviously, declared Rentoul, this was the promoters' true intention. If the protection of poor childbearing women had indeed been their chief object, their Bill would have provided for the tight control of midwives which was a feature of most Continental schemes, including local supervision, penalties for midwives exceeding the prescribed limits of their task, and the prohibition of unqualified practice. Without such restrictions, registration would give midwives a false idea of their own competence and importance, and the only result of registering them would be the very opposite of the promoters' predictions—namely, an enormous increase in baby-farming, criminal abortions, still-births and maternal deaths.

Basic to the registrationists' case had been the contention that a large proportion of childbearing women could not afford the doctor's fee. This 'notion' Dr. Rentoul contemptuously dismissed, claiming that it had only arisen because the West End consultants supporting the Bill believed that a doctor should never charge less than two guineas. Yet plenty of well-qualified young doctors were willing to take as little as 7s. 6d. to 10s. 6d. Moreover, if a family could not afford the doctor's fee in the first place, how could they pay him when, acting in accordance with the Bill's requirements, the registered midwife called him in to an emergency? He was sick of all this 'cant' about poverty; if the working-class smoked and drank less, they could easily pay the doctor.

However, women who *genuinely* could not afford the fee should be attended by the Poor Law Medical Officer. Here Dr. Rentoul took the opportunity of attacking those Guardians who employed midwives at a few shillings a case, rather than their Medical Officer at the prescribed Poor Law rates of 10s. to £2, or who required him to perform this work without extra payment. However, Rentoul's argument ignored the well-known reluctance of many Guardians to grant an order for their Medical Officer's attendance, and further, the unwillingness of some Medical Officers to undertake the work.[11] His criticisms of lying-in hospitals and charities for employing midwives left similar realities out of account. His suggestion that these institutions should only employ medical men was not likely to commend itself to their managers, perennially faced with financial problems, and in any case conscious that their patients' maternal death-rate usually compared very favourably with that reported by the Registrar-General for the nation at large.[12]

Rentoul's assertion that there were many 'well-qualified' young doctors willing to attend midwifery cases for as little as 7s. 6d. to 10s. 6d. (fees which would compete with those charged by many midwives) was promptly challenged by the *Lancet*.[13] Indeed, a contemporary manual for the young man entering general practice recommended a charge of not less than a guinea for ordinary midwifery,[14] and it is likely that lower fees were only acceptable as part of the cheaper contract practice undertaken by younger men working in poorer urban areas. In this period, as in earlier ones, midwifery was valued as the way into family practice, but as soon as this was firmly established, only the more lucrative cases would be taken, the rest being relinquished as exhausting, time-consuming, and furnishing only a poor financial return compared with other branches of medicine. The doctor in Bartley's *Village Pauper* charged a guinea even for wives of farm labourers on 15s. a week, and this, he declared, did not pay him for the travelling and waiting entailed by such attendance. Indeed, a common selling point in contemporary advertisements for the sale of medical practices was that a comfortable income (approximately £400–£650 a year) could be obtained without midwifery, or with none under a guinea or two guineas. What proportion of practitioners continued throughout life to depend on cheap midwifery for a sizeable part of their income is difficult to determine, though it is likely that their numbers were considerable. Certainly many doctors were glad to give up such work altogether when the 1911 national insurance scheme gave them an assured income for the first time.

It was precisely these poorer practitioners whose interests were likely to be ignored by the established leaders of the profession—the hospital consultants or affluent general practitioners—in London or the provinces. Part of the medical Establishment was, of course, the General Medical Council, which had twice voted for registration. Now that body, too, came under Dr. Rentoul's fire. It was their neglect of midwifery instruction in the medical curriculum, he argued, which had made it possible for midwives to claim that their training was better than that of many medical men.[15] Insisting that he was not against the better training of midwives, but only against their registration, Rentoul nevertheless urged that the improvement of midwifery instruction for medical students should take priority, there not being enough training material for both groups.

Supporters of registration had pointed favourably to the example of Continental countries. For Dr. Rentoul, however, their example served as a solemn warning of the dangers registration could hold for the English practitioner. On the Continent midwives might be allowed to vaccinate, attend abnormal births, and use instruments. Ultimately this would happen in England, since the Midwives' Institute would not rest satisfied with the provisions of the present Bill. Registration would thus create an inferior order of practitioners, which would not only rob the general practitioner of midwifery, but —subsidized by the State after the Continental pattern—might one day supersede the public vaccinator and the Poor Law Medical Officer. The Institute's real object, Rentoul contended, was to gain for women access to medical practice through a back door, thus increasing the competition already suffered by the 'over-stocked' profession from the prescribing chemist, the unqualified practitioner, and the quack. Reversing the old medical argument that if women wanted to enter the medical field they should rest content with being midwives, Rentoul insisted that women wishing to practise midwifery should take the full medical curriculum. The old apothecary had gone; now the ancient midwife should be replaced by the lady doctor.

Finally, if midwives were registered, registration for nurses would surely follow. It would then be difficult to resist the claim of the unqualified assistant and the prescribing chemist—both classes who were also largely relied on by the public. There was no real demand for registration, either from the medical profession or the country. The campaign for the Bill was merely a conspiracy between leading consultants who wished to 'dictate' to the general practitioner, and the women's rights movement who wanted to extend women's employment. The Bill marked a crisis for the medical profession and should be opposed with all the strength the profession could muster.

Dr. Rentoul himself was actively seeking support for his views among the membership of the B.M.A. At the Association's Annual Meeting in July he read a paper opposing registration and succeeded in having a motion passed calling for a delay on the Bill. The correspondence columns of the *British Medical Journal* and the *Lancet* showed that he was not alone in his opinions, and the *Provincial Medical Journal* called on its readers to lobby their M.P.s against the Bill. However, the enthusiasm with which Rentoul pressed his views did not always commend him to the local branches of the Association.

Advocates of registration were quick to answer the criticisms of Rentoul and his supporters. Dealing with the complaint that registration would create a 'new order of practitioners', they pointed out that midwives already enjoyed legal recognition, in that they could recover fees in a court of law. Far from building up the midwife into a quasi-medical practitioner, registration would place limits on her practice and restrict her to attendance on natural labour.[16] On the proposal that women who could not afford the doctor's fee should be attended by the Poor Law Medical Officer, registrationists took their stand on the Victorian principle of the superiority of self-help. Their intention was to provide poor women with safe midwifery attendance at a price they could afford, a policy, they argued, which had the great virtue of inculcating in the poor 'a proper feeling of independence', rather than encouraging increased reliance on the rates, already quite high enough.[17]

At the B.M.A. Annual Meeting, it had been maintained by Dr. Aveling that the profession generally favoured registration. However, some registrationists agreed in part with Dr. Rentoul's criticisms of the amended Bill, and supported his call for delay. Though regarding the amended Bill as a great improvement on the original, the *Lancet* was much concerned that disciplinary matters had been left to the Privy Council, and that there was no local machinery to exercise what it called 'proper discipline' over midwives. Some critics were strongly opposed to County Councils being required to undertake any of these tasks, holding that uniformity of standards would never be achieved with 132 different examining bodies, especially as ultimate responsibility would lie with laymen. The Council of the Obstetrical Society in particular felt that the 'politicians' of the Privy Council had snubbed them in ignoring their well-known views on the desirability of a small number of specially constituted medical boards for all duties pertaining to registration.[18]

Moreover, many supporters of registration, including the Midwives' Institute itself, shared Dr. Rentoul's doubts on the wisdom of initially allowing on to the register untrained midwives who were in 'bona fide' practice. They refused to accept Dr. Aveling's assurance that such women would not bother to enrol, and like Dr. Rentoul pointed to the Dentists and Veterinary Surgeons Acts as a warning of what might happen. Under these measures many ignorant and incompetent persons (including some not actually in practice at all) had been allowed to register as existing practitioners. This problem was likely to prove greater with midwives than it had with dentists, since the number of women eligible for registration, though a matter of dispute, was without doubt greater.[19]

Hitherto the campaign against the Bill had been undertaken entirely by general practitioners. Early in 1891, however, they were joined by the well known obstetrician Loombe Atthill, representative of the Irish College of Physicians on the G.M.C. As ex-Master of the Rotunda Hospital, Atthill had considerable experience of midwife training, and his opposition added considerable weight to the movement against the Bill. Atthill was not against the improvement of midwives, however, but only against their registration. It was his opinion, as it was still Florence Nightingale's,[20] that the provision of adequate training facilities was the first and most important step. This should be followed by provision for close and efficient supervision of midwife practice, without which the registered midwife would grow conceited with her new-found status and prove more dangerous than her untrained predecessor. The only solution was to provide the poor with trained and salaried midwives through the establishment of a network of maternity charities on lines similar to the Irish dispensary system. There was no registration in Ireland, and if England would only follow the Irish example, efficient and well-conducted midwives would soon be found all over the country.[21]

Yet during all this discussion of the Bill's probable results, all parties were ignorant of the extent of midwife practice. Nobody knew how many midwives there were, or whether they would bother to register. Like Atthill, some thought that registration would be popular, and would encourage large numbers of women to take up the work. But if, as Aveling expected, only a few enrolled, it would be a long time before the Act had any noticeable effect. Further, if poor mothers were to continue to prefer the cheaper Gamp, registration unaccompanied by the provision of a free or subsidized trained midwife service would be of no benefit to them.

Meanwhile the promoters' hopes that their Bill would be debated in the new session had been disappointed. By now there were demands from both friends and opponents for a Parliamentary enquiry into the whole subject, and both sides had applied to the Lord President, Lord Cranbrook, requesting a Select Committee. But despite the willingness of his department the year before to draft its own Bill, the Lord President was now far from enthusiastic, declaring himself unable to support a Bill on which the medical profession was so divided, and which did not protect poor mothers by preventing the practice of the unqualified woman. In any case, the improvement of midwives, like that of nurses, might well be achieved without resort to legislation. Although agreeing with the suggestion of a Select Committee, he considered that there were too many difficulties in the way of setting one up that year.

Late in April Mr. Pease bowed to the general feeling in favour of a Select Committee, and withdrew his Bill. The opposition was growing fast. *The Medical Press and Circular*, which had earlier welcomed the Bill, was now castigating the B.M.A. for having approved proposals to create 'another Frankenstein to gobble up the hapless general practitioner'.[22] But the promoters had suffered a more severe set-back than this. Sir Walter Foster, who had backed the original Bill and defended the amended version at the B.M.A.'s Annual Meeting the previous July, had now defected to the enemy. At this year's Annual Meeting he condemned the Bill as a 'hopeless attempt at legislation', and announced that he would oppose any future measure which did not have the approval of his 'medical brethren'. But despite this access of support, Dr. Rentoul and his supporters still failed to persuade the Annual Meeting to declare outright opposition to midwife legislation.

Sir Walter's conversion was without doubt connected with his desire for re-election to the G.M.C. the following December. Early in the year all three of the profession's direct representatives had received a clear warning from the *Provincial Medical Journal* that their re-election would be opposed if they supported the Bill, and both Sir Walter and Mr. Wheelhouse had given the anti-registrationists the assurances they sought. Dr. Glover, however, who along with Sir Walter had called for legislation in the G.M.C. two years before, stood firm.

But these three were not the only candidates in the election. Late in the day two new men, Mr. George Brown, a general practitioner in Bloomsbury, and Dr. Frederick Alderson, in general practice in Hammersmith, announced their candidature. Both had been put forward by the new General Practitioners' Union, formed by Brown (a founder of the Medical Defence Union) a few months before. Brown saw the new association as the champion of the ordinary medical man, whose interests in his view had too long been neglected by the recognized spokesmen of the profession. Among the Union's objects were an increase in direct representation of the profession on the G.M.C. (in particular of general practice), an end to the 'abuse' of medical charities, the prohibition of unqualified medical practice, and the defeat of that latest threat to the general practitioner, the Midwives Bill. But although midwife registration thus became the test issue in the election, it was Dr. Glover, the only candidate who still unequivocally favoured it, who topped the poll, the new candidates coming last. However, the degree of support which the latter had received was sufficient to encourage their backers to look forward with confidence to the next election in five years' time.

In the meantime a useful ally had been gained in Mrs. Bedford Fenwick and her *Nursing Record*. Ever since the 1890 Bill had been published, anti-midwife interests had been wooing the nurses' movement in the hope of gaining support for their opposition to midwife legislation. Mrs. Fenwick, flattered by their approval of the line taken by the *Record* on the Midwives Bill, had allowed leading opponents generous space in that journal. She herself was now beginning to talk about 'ending' the midwife. Midwives were a dangerous 'anachronism', who were doomed in the natural evolution of things soon to disappear, replaced by the better-educated and more efficient 'obstetric nurse' working under medical supervision. The title of 'Midwife' would thus become no more than a 'historical curiosity'.[23]

In the meantime the British Nurses' Association was making another attempt to gain statutory powers to register nurses—and nurse-midwives—this time applying to the Board of Trade for a licence of registration as a limited company. However, there was considerable hostility to the Association's plan. Opposition came from a large number of organizations and individuals in the hospital and nursing worlds, including the Midwives' Institute, and the doyenne of nursing, Florence Nightingale. In consequence the Association's petition was refused, on the grounds that its proposed scheme was not adequate for the satisfactory execution of its objects.

After this failure, the *Record* became even more abusive towards the Midwives' Institute, and particularly towards its Treasurer, Miss Rosalind Paget. Angered by the 'animus' which she alleged the Institute had shown towards nurse registration, Mrs. Fenwick now openly aligned herself with the Institute's enemies, hoping thereby to advance her own cause. For the next ten years she was to do all in her power to hinder the registration of midwives, giving up the fight only just in time to accept defeat with a good grace.

Mrs. Fenwick was not alone in looking forward to the time when all midwives should have nurse training. However, her confidence in the speedy disappearance of the 'midwife pure and simple' was completely unrealistic at that time. Again, in urging that the care of all lying-in women should be in the hands of a doctor, aided by a trained nurse, she was advocating something which could only be generally guaranteed by a free public midwifery service—not to be available until the advent of the National Health Service in 1948.

But if 1891 had not been a good year for the progress of Mrs. Fenwick's cause, neither had the supporters of midwife registration made much headway. It was not until May of the following year that a Select Committee of the Commons was appointed to enquire into the need for the improvement and registration of midwives. Fortunately for the registration party the Committee included several of its supporters, and was chaired by Mr. Fell Pease, the promoter of the 1890 Bill. However, a few weeks later came the General Election which brought the Liberals back to power, and it was not until the summer of 1893 that the Committee was reappointed and produced its final report.

Altogether, twenty-seven persons had appeared before the Committee,[24] and only five had opposed registration. Medical witnesses in favour included leading obstetricians, Medical Officers of Health, coroners, a Poor Law Medical Officer, general practitioners and women doctors. Dr. James Edmunds, still prepared to argue for the registration of educated lady midwives as a separate class, also gave evidence. Among other supporters were representatives of the Midwives' Institute, the Workhouse Infirmary Nursing Association, the Queen's Jubilee Nursing Institute, and other nursing associations.

Several witnesses drew unfavourable comparisons between the position of English midwives and that of midwives on the Continent, and even of midwives in India, where the Government had instituted free training schemes. Instances were quoted of death and injury to mother and child resulting from the midwife's incompetence, and Dr. Aveling went so far as to claim that eight mothers a day were 'sacrificed' to the ignorance of untrained women. The two coroners giving evidence emphasized that some midwives actively connived at the child's death, often burying as still-born children who had been born alive. In consequence most witnesses expected a striking reduction in maternal and infant mortality to follow an increase in the number of trained midwives. The trained midwife, they argued, would be greatly superior in her care for the safety and comfort of both mother and child—a matter of increasing public concern on account of the lower birth-rate, which had fallen from its peak of over 36 per 1,000 of the population in 1876 to about 30 in 1889. Experience also showed that the trained woman was far more willing than her untrained counterpart to send when appropriate for the doctor. In addition she could take steps for the prevention of 'ophthalmia neonatorum', or blindness in the new-born, an affliction which could result from contamination of the child's eyes by infected secretions from the birth canal, and which had been estimated as accounting for about one-third of the population of blind asylums. It was also expected that trained women would be less likely to indulge in the 'evil practices' of abortion and child murder.

Some witnesses maintained that many poor women employed midwives because they preferred to be attended by a woman. Others thought that this was largely a matter of low income, especially as the midwife generally undertook nursing duties also. Most thought that the trained midwife would gradually come to be preferred to the unqualified woman, but that the medical profession had nothing to fear from registration, as midwives would only attend the poor. Indeed, the position of the medical man would be enhanced, since the trained midwife could relieve him of a great deal of arduous and ill-paid work.

Among the five opponents of registration was only one obstetrician. This was Loombe Atthill, whose objection was not to the improvement of midwives, but merely to their registration. The rest were men actively concerned in the new general practitioners' movement, and besides Rentoul and Brown, included Dr. Hugh Woods of Highgate, and Dr. Lovell Drage of Hatfield. These men took their stand on the 1886 Medical Act, arguing—wrongly, however—that it required all persons legally recognized as qualified to practise midwifery to possess qualifications in medicine and surgery also, and that midwife registration would in consequence contravene the Act.[25] The registered midwife would certainly harm the general practitioner, since she would rob him of the midwifery which was often the mainstay of his practice. Outside London, they claimed, the majority of the profession was strongly against registration, and although such provincial practitioners might seem very insignificant to the members of the 'superior' College of Physicians, who were supporting registration, their views deserved equal consideration.

Dr. Rentoul gave evidence at length, making use in the process of contradictory, and sometimes defamatory, statements. Arguing that midwives were unnecessary because there were plenty of well-qualified young doctors willing to attend the poor at no more than the midwife's fee, he at the same time complained that the midwifery training of many of these men was grossly deficient. While conceding that midwives were often better trained, he insisted that as 'uneducated' persons they must be more dangerous, mistakenly illustrating his contention with the fatal case of Princess Charlotte, George IV's daughter, who had, of course, been attended by a man.

In any case, Dr. Rentoul maintained, most women preferred a male attendant in childbirth. The few who wished to have a woman could, he thought, be attended by woman doctors—a proposal which ignored the fact that there were only about thirty practising in the whole country,[26] and that the poor could no more afford their fees than those of the male practitioner. Ridiculing as 'absurd' the very low maternal death-rates claimed by the well-known maternity charities, Dr. Rentoul alleged that such figures were arrived at only by 'cooking' the records. Furthermore, without the strict oversight of midwives which obtained in Prussia, an increase in trained women would bring a rise in criminal abortions and still-births. Since it was unlikely that Parliament would agree to institute a similar system of supervision in England, registration would merely create an 'independent order of practitioners' to the detriment of the profession and the public.

Dr. Rentoul was strongly supported in this line by Mr. George Brown and Dr. Hugh Woods of the General Practitioners' Union. Even more outspoken than Dr. Rentoul, they made it clear that they looked forward in the very near future to the total disappearance of the midwife. As a result of civilization, they argued, childbirth could no longer be regarded as a natural process, nor could 'natural' labour be accurately defined. Every birth should therefore be attended by a medical practitioner, who, said Dr. Woods, should not remain an 'idle spectator', but 'guide' and 'control' it after the modern American practice. Such attendance would be quite possible in the present 'full condition' of the medical profession, and poor women could be attended either free or for a 'small payment' from the State. Though midwives would no longer exist, there would be scope for women to work as monthly nurses, carrying out that part of the attendance more suitable for a 'mere woman'. In the meantime, an inquest should be held on every fatal case attended by a midwife, who should receive a 'sharp reprimand' from the coroner; midwife practice would then soon die out.

In August 1893, the Select Committee produced its report. Following the weight of the evidence before it, it recommended in favour of legislation to protect the title of the registered midwife, who, it concluded, would not injure the medical profession, but on the contrary relieve it of much 'irksome and ill-paid work'. The G.M.C. should be required to frame the rules governing examinations and discipline, which should be subject to the approval of the Privy Council, the County Councils being made responsible for local administration. The Report proposed increased facilities for midwife training in lying-in hospitals and in Poor Law infirmaries.[27] The Committee had not had the advice of the Local Government Board, which, despite the Guardians' continuing employment of midwives under the Poor Law, and in contrast to James Stansfield's active interest twenty years before, had declined the Committee's invitation to express an opinion.

The Committee had accepted the view that much unnecessary maternal and infant mortality was caused by the untrained midwife. At this time there was no system of notification of births, nor any statistics on the sex and qualifications of the attendant. Thus any attempt at quantifying this mortality, such as that made by Dr.

Aveling before the Committee, could only be the merest guess-work. Many births were attended neither by qualified practitioners, nor by midwives, trained or untrained, but by unqualified *men*. These were sometimes chemists, but some carried on trades quite unrelated to medicine. More usually, they were the unqualified assistants—often medical students, or failed medical students—of a registered practitioner. Such assistants might staff as many as fifteen or twenty dispensaries for their qualified principal, who generally attended their cases only when a death certificate was necessary.

However, as Dr. Farr had concluded in the Registrar-General's Annual Report for 1876, some avoidable mortality was clearly still attributable to the less skilful *registered* practitioner, a point which Dr. James Edmunds, outspoken as ever, had made to the Select Committee. Indeed, many of Aveling's fellow obstetricians did not share his confidence in the generally high level of medical performance in this field, and Dr. W. C. Grigg, Physician to Queen Charlotte's Lying-in Hospital, concluded that more cases of 'injury and physical disaster' resulted from the imprudent use of forceps and turning by medical men than from the negligence and ignorance of midwives. It was, of course, the old story. Under pressure from a busy practice, doctors often fell into the temptation of unduly expediting the birth.[28] In addition, despite the clear demonstration by leading lying-in hospitals over the last ten years of the value of antiseptics in childbirth, many practitioners refused to take them seriously.[29] According to Dr. W. S. Playfair, consultant to the General Lying-in Hospital, not one medical man in a hundred in private practice used antiseptics in any regular and systematic manner.[30]

For the supporters of registration the Report of the Select Committee was a great advance. That summer, too, it had been made clear that for the time being at least legal sanction would *not* be given to the British Nurses' Association (now granted the prefix 'Royal') to carry out its own scheme to register nurses, and along with them, midwives. After the failure in 1891 of its application to the Board of Trade, the Association had made another attempt to gain these powers, this time petitioning the Queen through the Privy Council for a Royal Charter. As before, the application had met with considerable opposition, including that of the Midwives' Institute. The signature of Florence Nightingale headed the counter-petition, and as a result of her influence behind the scenes, the Charter finally granted to the Association gave it no power to keep the statutory register it desired, but only a list with no official significance. Mrs. Fenwick put on a brave front, with talk of the 'State recognition of nursing' conferred by the Charter. But she had clearly been defeated, and was now forced to turn to other means to gain her ends. Although she had previously derided the Midwives' Institute for seeking 'that help of the helpless', an Act of Parliament,[31] it was not long before she herself was actively campaigning for a Nurses' Registration Act.

But the anti-midwife interests had also gained ground. As was to be expected, they challenged the Select Committee's Report, complaining that the enquiry had not been exhaustive enough, and that insufficient weight had been given to the views of the main body of the profession.[32] In the influential Metropolitan and Home Counties Branch of the B.M.A. the resolution passed in favour of registration on the occasion of Aveling's address in 1873 had been rescinded— a victory for George Brown's General Practitioners' Union. The Union had also acquired a cheap weekly, which, under the title of the *Medical Times and Hospital Gazette*, now joined the *Provincial Medical Journal* in a consistent anti-midwife line.

Besides this, the struggle had now been brought to the G.M.C. There, through the agency of Mr. C. G. Wheelhouse, one of the profession's direct representatives, Dr. Rentoul and his colleagues hoped to persuade the G.M.C. to withdraw its repeated statements in favour of midwife registration. Since a direct attack was impossible, the ploy used was to suggest that the certificates granted in ever-increasing numbers by midwife-training institutions could be mistaken by the public for medical diplomas, and that medical men signing them should be declared guilty of 'conduct infamous in a professional respect'.[33] If the G.M.C. could be persuaded to agree to this proposal, it would not only mean the end of hospital examinations and certificates, but also the end of the Obstetrical Society's examination, which, as the only independent one in the country, had already laid the basis for registration. This would, of course, strike the death-blow of the registration movement.

At first the G.M.C. dealt with Dr. Rentoul's complaint by merely rejecting it. Eighteen months later, however, in May 1894, he was more successful. The G.M.C. agreed to request institutions granting diplomas and certificates to midwives to ensure that these could not be confused with those issued by bodies legally recognized to grant medical qualifications. Although this concession did not give Dr. Rentoul all he had wanted, it still represented a tactical success for his campaign. It had shown how determined organization on the part of rank-and-file general practitioners could influence even the G.M.C.—a development of great importance for the future. Dr. Rentoul, when reviewing the achievement of the anti-registrationists during the last three and a half years, was justly able to claim that for such 'unimportant persons' this was 'not a bad "show" '.[34]

Indeed, the growing strength of the opposition indicated how far the B.M.A. had misjudged the feeling of many general practitioners on the midwife question. Before the 1890 Bill was introduced into Parliament, the *British Medical Journal* had been supremely confident that the whole profession favoured registration, and that it was only the 'plethora' of Parliamentary business which had prevented a Midwives Bill from being enacted.[35] But the challenge to B.M.A. leadership on midwives was not merely a criticism of its handling of this question alone; it was also an indication of the general dissatisfaction with the hierarchical organization of the Association itself, which was eventually to force its reconstitution in 1902 on more democratic lines.[36]

But medical opposition, though the most serious obstacle to midwife registration, was not the only one which its supporters had to face. Trained midwives were by no means unanimous in wanting a Midwives Act, and the nurse registration movement was allied with the midwife's bitterest enemies. There were lay opponents, too, who on principle condemned any extension of registration legislation, and who objected to proposals to place stricter requirements on midwives than were imposed by comparable legislation on the male professions. For all these reasons a midwives' registration Act had proved much more difficult to achieve than its advocates had first imagined, and it was now abundantly clear that wider public backing had to be obtained if there was to be any hope of success in the future.

CHAPTER SEVEN

State Register or Local Licence?

During the seven years which followed the report of the Select Committee of 1893 there were to be several unsuccessful attempts to secure the passage of a Midwives Bill into law, and successive Bills were put forward by the uneasy coalition of interests which advocated registration. These Bills differed widely in the degree of control to which it was proposed to subject midwives and the power to be accorded to the medical profession over the registration machinery, thus reflecting the varying weight of medical and lay influence among the promoters and the strength of medical pressure groups hostile to registration.

As in the past, opposition to registration came also from among midwives themselves. Many of them, along with a section of the women's rights movement, regarded any proposal to place midwives under medical control as yet another instance of the male medical imperialism from which women, both as patients and as workers, would inevitably suffer. But the most serious obstruction of all was to come from the militant group of general practitioners who represented the less affluent members of the profession. These men, far from desiring an enhancement of the midwife's status, wished to see her disappear altogether—a feasible aim, as North American experience has since shown. At the same time their continuing alliance with the nurses seeking registration widened the rift between the two groups of women working to raise the occupations of nursing and midwifery to the level of respectable employments for middle-class women.

So the struggle continued, making little or no impression upon the general public. Despite the predictions and counter-predictions of the embattled interests as to the likely effects of registration on maternal and infant mortality neither the 1892–96 Liberal Government, nor the Conservative administration which succeeded it, was prepared to help in bringing a Bill before Parliament. Yet the State had already taken decisive action on other questions of infant welfare. In 1891 a Tory Government had prohibited women from working in factories for a month after childbirth—a restriction on women's liberty strongly condemned by the defenders of women's rights and in the event unenforceable.[1] However, midwife registration, as John Simon had already pointed out, might well prove expensive to operate and raised other complicated issues. Thus it was not until national confidence in the physical capacity of the British race to sustain an imperial role had been sufficiently undermined by the defeats of the Boer War that the Conservative Government was willing to go as far as adopting even a benevolent neutrality in its approach to midwife legislation.

The account of the differences between the various groups advocating registration, and of their attempts to gain wider support for their changing proposals, is of necessity detailed and complex. For these reasons the general reader may prefer to turn to the following chapter, in which the story of the struggle for a Midwives Act is brought to a successful conclusion.

The favourable report of the 1893 Select Committee had been an important milestone on the road to legislation. The task now facing the different groups working for this object was not only to gain enough support in Parliament for their next Bill, but also to agree among themselves on what form it should take. Since the Select Committee had endorsed the Privy Council's views that examination and registration should be in the hands of local government there was a strong possibility that the next Bill would follow its recommendations, especially as there was at the time no medical body actively working for legislation. It was to frustrate this threat to medical control of the registration machinery that in the autumn of 1893 a group of medical men decided to form an association to work to influence the provisions of the next Bill. Dr. Aveling, hitherto the leader of the medical registrationists, had died of typhoid the year before, and the leaders of the new 'Midwives Registration Association' were two London practitioners, Mr. F. R. Humphreys, and Dr. R. Boxall, Visiting Physician to the General Lying-in Hospital. Appealing to their professional brethren for support, they warned them that legislation was inevitable; it was therefore vital that the medical point of view should be taken into account in the drafting of the next Bill. This appeal was not unsuccessful, and by October 1894 the Association could boast a membership of over 330 from all parts of the country and from every sphere of practice.

Meanwhile, the Midwives' Institute itself had not been idle. Mindful of anti-registrationist criticism that there had been no wide demand for legislation, the Institute set out to gain backing for a

Midwives Bill among the general and philanthropic public. Since Dr. Aveling had brought the question before the Social Science Association in 1874 there had been no public discussion of the issue by such bodies, or in the general press. Since this was indeed a 'woman's question', the first step was to mobilize the support of women, and more especially, of the women's political organizations whose growth had been such a feature of the past ten years.[2] For this a larger, more widely based pressure group was needed, which could take the campaign all over the country. Thus while Dr. Boxall and Mr. Humphreys were founding their association of medical men, the Institute was setting on foot a new women's organization, the 'Association for Promoting the Compulsory[3] Registration of Midwives'. Among the Association's leadership were influential Society ladies[4] and the wives of bishops and Members of Parliament, and before long it had gained the adherence of the Women's Co-operative Guild, the National Union of Women Workers, and the Women's Liberal Federation.

The opposition was also active. Though there was at the moment no Bill before the public, Dr. Rentoul was still indefatigably waging his campaign to persuade the G.M.C. to take action against medical men who examined midwives and awarded them certificates of qualification. Finally, in December 1894, his efforts—which had been directed principally against the Obstetrical Society's examination—met with success. Although the Society's diploma merely stated that its holder was a 'skilled midwife, competent to attend Natural Labour', and no evidence was produced to show that anyone had ever been misled into thinking that its holder was *medically* qualified, the G.M.C., to the Society's great surprise, declared it a 'colourable imitation' of a medical diploma.

However, this was not, as the anti-registration interests had hoped, the end of the examination and certification of midwives, and so of the registration movement. The G.M.C. had not been willing to go as far as Dr. Rentoul wished, and declare the certification of midwives 'unprofessional' conduct—indeed, it had no power to do so. Nor was the Obstetrical Society prepared to abandon its examination. Led by its President, Dr. F. W. Champneys, a dedicated worker for the improvement of midwives, and later first Chairman of the Central Midwives Board, the Society soon agreed with the G.M.C. to replace its diploma by a smaller and less impressive looking 'certificate'. The Society's work for midwives continued, and its qualification was sought by increasing numbers of midwives as each year passed.

At the same time the anti-midwife group had been consolidating its position by forming an alliance with the nurse registration movement. This had been achieved through the accession of Dr. Bedford Fenwick to the editorial staff of the *Medical Times*, the journal of the General Practitioners' Union, now re-named the Medical Practitioners' Association. Supporting the Rentoul line, Mrs. Fenwick kept up her barrage against midwife registration in her *Nursing Record*. By bolstering up an 'obsolete' class of women, doomed to be superseded under the unalterable law of the survival of the fittest by the three-year trained 'obstetric nurse',[5] the Obstetrical Society had betrayed its medical brethren. No thoroughly trained nurse, Mrs. Fenwick told her readers, could support this attempt to raise to professional status such 'untrained and ignorant workers'.[6]

Early in 1895 the two Associations working for registration came together to promote a new Bill, setting up a 'Midwives Bill Committee' to draft it. The Committee included sympathetic M.P.s, both lay and medical, eminent London obstetricians, representatives of the Midwives' Institute and of the London Lying-in Hospitals, and Henry Burdett, Secretary of the Hospitals' Association. The Chairman was a leading Conservative peer, Lord Balfour of Burleigh, whose able advocacy was to do much to give the campaign status in the public eye.

The resultant Bill was a testimony to the predominant influence of the medical men of the Midwives Registration Association. A clause explicitly restricting the midwife to attendance on natural labour was reinstated, despite the Privy Council's objections to its inclusion in the 1890 Bill. The midwife's right of appeal to the Privy Council, also a proposal of that body, was dispensed with. However, in consequence of Bradlaugh's earlier opposition the clause requiring that practising midwives should all produce evidence of good character before admission to the register, had been abandoned.

Medical influence showed itself again in the proposal to place the registration machinery solely under medical control. Examinations were to be conducted by local medical boards, appointed not by County Councils, but by the G.M.C., and responsible to a Central Board, which was also to deal with registration and discipline. The duty of reporting complaints against midwives was to be laid on Medical Officers of Health, or (to provide for counties with no such Officer) other medical practitioners appointed by the local health authority. These were, however, to be paid by the Central Board. Despite John Simon's earlier warnings on this point, there was no provision to finance the registration machinery other than by midwives' examination and registration fees. The Central Board itself was again to be a purely medical body, this time comprising three medical men chosen by the Midwives' Institute and three from each of the three London medical corporations. But although the Institute's representatives were to occupy a quarter of the seats on the Board—an improvement from their point of view on the 1890 Bill—medical interests were still to predominate, and there was to be no direct representation of midwives themselves.

Uneasy about this situation, the Institute called for the addition of three lay members, to be nominated by the Privy Council to represent the public interest. Yet its strong philanthropic motivation would not allow it to oppose the Bill on the issue of midwife representation. Reminding members that in past discussions on registration the Institute had consistently put aside its own interests, its secretary, Mrs. Margaret Nichol, urged that if there was any chance of legislation to protect poor lying-in mothers from the Gamp it would be wrong to hinder its passage into law. 'Unlike some general practitioners', declared Mrs. Nichol, the Institute felt bound to look at the question from the standpoint of the public good, and in *Nursing Notes* she called on its members to support this position.[7]

The Bill was published early in May. It was immediately attacked by Dr. Rentoul, as even more 'dangerous and misleading' than the previous one, and designed with the sole aim of creating a new order of medical practitioners.[8] The *Lancet* was conciliatory, while the *Hospital* gave it general approval. Both journals warned the profession that it must not allow its own selfish interests to stand in the way of the public good, the *Hospital* pointing out that under the Bill the duties of the midwife would be limited and defined 'with the utmost possible strictness', and that registered medical practitioners would be 'absolute masters and judges' over her. However, the absence of a clause forbidding the practice of the unqualified woman was a serious deficiency.[9]

The *British Medical Journal* in general was cool, concentrating its fire on the 'extraordinary' proposal that the duty of reporting complaints against midwives to the Central Board should be laid on Medical Officers of Health.[10] But though the reason given was that this would be an invidious task for these officers, most of whom were in local private practice, it is more than likely that the general practitioners' fear of the growing importance of the Medical Officer of Health was an important factor in the journal's attitude. The Society of Medical Officers of Health, however, refused to commit themselves.

Mrs. Bedford Fenwick, as could be expected, had her own criticisms of the Bill. A keen supporter of women's rights, she pointed out that although it recognized the midwife as an independent practitioner, it placed her in the power of an entirely medical Board. This, she felt, was something which would be condemned by all 'self-respecting trained Midwives'—that is, the midwives who were also trained nurses whom she was hoping to attract to her project of nurse registration. But although opposing the Bill, Mrs. Fenwick was quick to extract the maximum advantage for her own cause. If 'ignorant women' were to be registered, she urged, it was vital that trained nurses should have their own Act, in order that they might be distinguished from women who were 'only' midwives.[11]

On 18 May 1895, the Bill was debated in the Lords, passing its second reading without a division. Speaking for the Government (Lord Rosebery's Liberal administration) Lord Playfair expressed the general approval of the Privy Council, but indicated that the department had various amendments in view. In the meantime, at the request of the Lord President, the G.M.C. had also considered the Bill. Yet despite strenuous efforts by its anti-midwife members to persuade their colleagues to demand further limitations on the registered midwife, it had proposed only minor amendments.

However, when the Bill reached its Committee stage in the Lords a few days later, it had been radically altered. In accordance with the views of the Privy Council, the medical control so important to the medical registrationists had been materially cut down. Local examination boards were now to be placed under the Central Board rather than under the G.M.C., and, as the Midwives' Institute had hoped, the Board's membership was to be increased by three persons appointed by the Crown to represent the public interest. Moreover, there was the novel condition that at least one of these members should be a *woman*, a requirement which made it possible for a midwife actually to sit on the Board which was to govern the recruitment and practice of her profession. Finally, the clause restricting the registered midwife to attendance on natural labour was again taken out to be incorporated in the rules.

Medical interests had thus lost considerable ground in the new version of the Bill. Not only was there no explicit restriction of the midwife to attendance on natural labour, but the proposed Central Midwives Board now appeared as a Frankenstein's monster, claiming life and independence of its own. The Board was now to appoint its own examiners, and would itself administer the regulations governing midwife practice. These powers, the *British Medical Journal* complained, would endow it in the eyes of the public with the same status as the G.M.C.—'a condition of things which, of course, has only to be mentioned to be condemned'.[12]

But although the Bill had made great progress, the time for a Midwives Act had not yet arrived. That same month Lord Rosebery's government fell, and in the election that followed the Conservatives were returned to power. The Bill accordingly lapsed, and although in the following year (1896) the promoters were successful in the private members' ballot, the Government took the day for its own business and discussion of the Bill was once more deferred.

In the meantime the power of the anti-midwife interests was growing, and at the B.M.A.'s Annual Meeting in July 1895 the group gained the victory which they had sought for several years. With the threat of Lord Balfour's Bill before the gathering, the opponents of registration had secured the passage of a resolution condemning midwife legislation. Moved by an important new adherent to the opposition, the distinguished gynaecologist Lawson Tait, the resolution declared its approval for any 'practical' scheme of nurse registration, while condemning any measure which had as its object the 'formation' of any class of independent practitioners not recognized by the 1886 Medical Act.

During the following months a number of other proposals for dealing with midwife regulation were laid before the profession. Among these was a scheme put forward by Dr. Rentoul himself. This would have outlawed all independent midwife practice, but would have registered women who worked as 'obstetric nurses' under medical direction.[13] Others put forward less stringent proposals which, though allowing for the legal recognition of the independent midwife, at the same time were designed to put her under extremely tight medical control. One such was canvassed by the B.M.A.'s Lancashire and Cheshire branch (Dr. Rentoul's own branch), which, besides calling midwives 'obstetric nurses', aimed to put them well into the power of local practitioners, and provided for any infringement of the Central Board's rules to be punished in a court of law. Yet another proposal, drawn by a Dr. Fraser of Salford, was for simple licensing of trained midwives by the local public health authority. Finally, the B.M.A. produced its own scheme. In deference to the opposition to midwife registration shown by many of its members at the previous Annual Meeting, this was described as a Midwifery Nurses Bill, though the women it proposed to register were still to be midwives in independent practice. In contrast to Lord Balfour's amended Bill, under the B.M.A. scheme the membership of the Central Board was to be completely medical and its doings firmly under G.M.C. control.[14]

Naturally, those who wanted to see the end of the midwife were not taken in by this effort to sugar the pill of registration. Condemning the B.M.A. for even considering legislation, they protested that its 'Midwifery Nurses Bill' was an unjustifiable attempt to mislead the profession; it was a Bill to register midwives and should be opposed as such. Mrs. Fenwick's *Nursing Record* supported this line, joining with the *Medical Times* in arguing for the registration of all nurses, including 'obstetric nurses', under 'medical control'. This, argued the *Record*, would solve the midwife problem satisfactorily for both the medical and nursing professions.[15]

In fact Mrs. Fenwick was in need of allies. Despite the resolution supporting nurse registration passed at the B.M.A. Annual Meeting the summer before, the opposition had proved too strong. The following January the B.M.A. Council had called a meeting of nursing organization representatives to consider the question. Two members of the Midwives' Institute, Miss Jane Wilson and Miss Katherine Twining, and Henry Burdett, Mrs. Fenwick's old enemy, had been present, and Dr. and Mrs. Fenwick had been outvoted. Moreover, the Fenwicks had recently been ousted from control of the Royal British Nurses' Association, and later in the year that body, founded expressly by Mrs. Fenwick to fight for nurse registration, resolved against it.

Furthermore, although many medical men opposed midwife legislation, this did not mean that they therefore supported the registration of nurses. To some of these the 'lady' nurse with her professional aspirations was as great a threat as the educated midwife. The whole nursing sisterhood, complained one medical critic, was too much 'pampered and petted'. The 'modern' nurse, 'with her grand get-up, her waist belt with a surgical instrument-maker's shop dangling to it, and her array of temperature charts and thermometers', was losing the capacity for 'real hard work and genuine nursing', and the 'real and proper' relationship between nurse and doctor was in danger of being lost.[16] At the same time, employers of the private nurse protested that she was 'too educated and high-class' to fit into the household, and that she would not eat with the servants.[17] Such people were not going to join a movement which aimed at raising the nurse's position still further through state registration.

Mrs. Fenwick continued to fight. The registration of nurses, she argued, was of greater importance to the country than that of midwives, who would soon disappear. Indeed, the 'obstetric nurse', as she called the nurse-midwife, was everywhere replacing that 'strange survival of the unfit', the midwife pure and simple, and contrary to the views of 'arm-chair theorists' these well trained women were willing to work among the poor for the small fees they could offer.[18] This claim was, however, an exaggeration. Although, largely as a result of the efforts of the Queen's Nursing Institute, there was a steady increase in the supply of trained women practising in rural areas, these worked mainly as salaried employees of nursing associations. In other cases, patients' fees merely supplemented a private income. In her first year as a midwife in rural Somerset Miss

Alice Gregory (later a notable figure in the midwifery world) charged her patients 5s. per case, receiving only £27 10s. in all from her practice. Her main source of income was an allowance of £50 per annum from her father, the Dean of St. Paul's.[19]

In fact country posts in isolated country villages were not popular, and the salaries paid by nursing associations, which were no more than those to be commanded by an upper servant, were no great inducement. By 1896 the Queen's Institute itself had been forced to start training a class of 'Village Nurses', with only six months' instruction, who would live in their native villages and act as nurse-midwives.[20] This more practical approach had been adopted from its foundation in 1889 by the Plaistow Maternity Charity, which trained village women who were financed by 'benevolent ladies' or nursing associations. Indeed, it was a principle with Miss Katherine Twining, the Charity's Superintendent and founder, that the only solution to the problem of improving midwife practice in the country was not to aim at supplanting 'Sairey Gamp', but at transforming her.[21]

But even if educated women *had* been willing to settle in the country as midwives they were often not welcomed by the medical men of the area. Many of these were quick to resent the 'lady nurse' who on certain subjects might know more than they, and despite agreements between her nursing association and local medical men that she would only attend the poor, she was often regarded as a competitor, on account of her lower fees.[22] Alice Gregory had to promise local medical men that she would not attend the wives of tradesmen, clerks, farmers or firemen, or any woman who had previously been attended by a doctor, without the latter's sanction.[23] The hostility felt by many general practitioners towards the trained midwife was summed up in a letter to the *British Medical Journal* from an angry Mortlake practitioner, Dr. McCook Weir. The professional nurse 'with her thermometer and her tongue', protested Dr. McCook Weir, was bad enough, but the certificated midwife was an 'outrage' against the medical practitioner.[24]

Over and above this medical hostility, the new trained midwife might have to contend with the indifference of the poor whom she had been appointed to serve. Nursing associations often had difficulty in persuading mothers that it was no part of the midwife's duty to cook or clean for the family, as the untrained woman often did. Besides this, many women felt more comfortable being attended by a neighbour, who—like the Mrs. Quinton recalled by Flora Thompson in *Lark Rise to Candleford*, was poor like themselves. Unlike the trained midwives who came later, she was no 'superior person' coming into the household to strain its resources to the utmost, or shame her patients into forced confessions of what they lacked for the occasion.

In his letter to the *British Medical Journal* Dr. McCook Weir had predicted that a Midwives Act, although the ambition of every 'ladies' committee' in the land, would never reach the Statute Book. Yet in the past two years the registration movement had gained greatly in strength, largely as a result of the work of such 'ladies' committees'. The Association for the Compulsory Registration of Midwives now had ten local branches, and a membership of two thousand among women of all classes.

But the opposition had also gained ground. Mr. George Brown, President of the Medical Practitioners' Association and editor of the *Medical Times*, was now a member of the B.M.A. Parliamentary Bills Committee, and was thus in a good position to influence the Association's midwife policy. More important, both Brown and Rentoul were candidates in the forthcoming G.M.C. election, in which neither Mr. Wheelhouse nor Sir Walter Foster were seeking re-election. Both were successful, with Dr. Glover, still steadfast in his support of registration, coming a poor third.

Quick to congratulate the new members in her *Nursing Record*, Mrs. Fenwick hailed their victory as proof that the whole medical profession was against midwife legislation.[25] Since, as on the previous occasion, only about a third of the electorate had voted, this was clearly an exaggeration. What the election *had* shown, however, was how effective a small but organized group of general practitioners could be. Above all, it had clearly demonstrated that the next Midwives Bill would meet an opposition even more effective and dangerous than before.

Early in 1897 the new Bill appeared. Based on the 1896 version, it included some important additions and amendments which had as their object an increase in the power to be exercised over midwives by the medical profession, and thus represented a swing in favour of medical interests. Though the composition of the Central Board remained the same, its rules were now to be approved by the G.M.C., with appeal to the Privy Council in cases of disagreement. Greater medical control at the local level was to be achieved by extending the duties of the Medical Officer of Health to include 'general supervision' of the midwives in his area in accordance with the rules to be laid down under the provisions of the Act. The Bill thus proposed a system of local medical inspection after the Prussian pattern so admired by Dr. Aveling in his *English Midwives* twenty-four years before.[26]

But the Bill contained another interesting and important innovation, which was to be included in all subsequent Midwives Bills and which is a feature of the latest measure of midwife regulation, the Midwives Act of 1951. Previous Bills had proposed that midwives, like doctors and dentists, should be liable to erasure from the register for convictions in a court of law, and for 'professional' misconduct. In the case of midwives, however, 'professional' misconduct would include the infringement of the comprehensive and detailed rules of practice to be laid down by the Central Midwives Board. Now, under this new provision, a midwife might also be struck off for 'other' *undefined* misconduct.[27] She would therefore be at risk if *any* aspect of her private life failed to meet with the approbation of the local Medical Officer of Health and of the Central Board, whose decision could only be appealed against by expensive legal action in the High Court. Thus midwives were expected to conform to a stricter standard of morality than male professions. Yet, far from objecting to this discrimination against women, the Midwives Institute seems positively to have welcomed the scope it gave for removing from the register those whose morals did not accord with its own narrow middle-class ideas of acceptable female behaviour.[28]

Unfortunately for the promoters, their Bill had secured only a low place in the Private Members' ballot, and as a result it was not debated that year. At the same time the B.M.A., under pressure from members urging severer restrictions on midwives than those proposed by the Bill before Parliament, and from militants like Brown, who opposed legislation of any kind, had been amending its own measure. Under the new title of 'Obstetric Nurses Registration Bill', this now avoided all mention of the word 'midwife', and included several features of the Lancashire and Cheshire branch's more stringent draft. It also contained a clause to prohibit practice by the unqualified woman, a provision which Dr. Rentoul had from the very first insisted was essential to any Bill really intended to protect the public.

Though there was to be no machinery for local supervision, the all-medical Central Board (appointed by the G.M.C.) was to consist of medical practitioners representing different parts of the country. All teachers and examiners of midwives (i.e. those leading obstetricians and members of the Obstetrical Society Council who generally favoured the improvement of midwives, and had experience in training them) were to be excluded. The midwife was thus to be firmly placed in the power of the rural general practitioner who so commonly viewed her as a competitor for practice he considered rightly his. As the Midwives' Institute commented, the spider was being invited to legislate for the fly.[29]

In the meantime Dr. Rentoul, now a newly elected member of the G.M.C., was embarking on an energetic campaign to enlist support for his own scheme to ban the independent midwife. This proposed that in all cases where the patient could not afford the doctor's fee, the Poor Law authorities should be required to provide her with a doctor, paid at 40s. the case, and a trained district nurse. Such a step, urged Rentoul, would be in the national interest, since the success of Britain as a colonial power demanded an expanding population.[30] But although this reversion to the eighteenth-century view of population growth was becoming more general, as yet its implications for the provision of public health services were not widely accepted. Any extension of the Poor Law Medical Service, the *Lancet* considered, would be open to the 'formidable' objection that it would lead to the 'pauperization' of the patient, while the Midwives' Institute ridiculed Rentoul's proposal as one to support medical men out of the rates.[31]

However, Dr. Rentoul's attempts to gain backing for his 'Obstetric Nurses Bill' were having little success, and in the middle of 1897, in what turned out to be his last major effort on the midwife question, he extended his proposals to include the registration of medical and surgical nurses.[32] Shortly afterwards, piqued by the lack of support, financial and otherwise, which he had received from the profession in his efforts to secure the promotion of his Bill, he resigned from the G.M.C., after only seven months' service. From now on Rentoul was to leave the fight against midwife registration largely to others.

In the ensuing G.M.C. election, the vacant seat was won by a young surgeon, Victor Horsley. A forceful and aggressive character, Horsley was already a leading figure in the B.M.A. Parliamentary Bills Committee. He was also President of the Medical Defence Union, an organization which had undertaken the prosecution of unqualified persons contravening the Apothecaries Act, and which was committed to seeking the amendment of the Medical Acts to allow the prohibition of all unqualified medical practice. Horsley supported legislation for midwives solely as a means of controlling them; he was thus to make a useful addition to the anti-midwife group on the G.M.C.

The following February the Midwives Bill was reintroduced into the Commons, and this time its chances appeared much stronger. Its sponsor was the Lord Advocate for Scotland, J. B. Balfour, a fact which, as the *British Medical Journal* commented, would of itself bring considerable support. Since Mr. Balfour had won first place in the ballot, the Bill could not be blocked as it had been the year before; the profession had therefore to act quickly if it wished to influence its provisions.[33]

In addition, the Bill's supporters were gaining some favourable publicity. The following month the influential *Contemporary Review* published an article by Dr. C. J. Cullingworth, Physician to the General Lying-in Hospital, which provided the first real discussion of the subject in the general press. Arguing that the incompetence of ignorant midwives was the cause of much unnecessary mortality, Cullingworth disabused his readers of the widely held notion that midwives attended only a very small proportion of births.[34] The lesson of the article was clear. To a nation beginning once more to be concerned about the size of its population, maternal and infant mortality were of great importance. If, as Cullingworth estimated, midwives attended as many as half or three-quarters of all births, the regulation of their practice was a matter of far more moment than had hitherto been supposed.

Under pressure from its militants, the B.M.A. had finally included a clause to prohibit unqualified practice in its own draft Bill. It was thus free to attack the measure before Parliament for reproducing the 'glaring defects' of the Medical Acts, which Horsley hoped to see similarly amended before long.[35] On the subject of local supervision of midwives, the B.M.A. was still opposed to its being undertaken by Medical Officers of Health, on the grounds that in large districts they would find the work too onerous, while in small ones they would not be sufficiently independent of local pressures.[36] The Society of Medical Officers of Health, however, raised no objection, provided that the work was adequately remunerated.[37]

The *Lancet* described the Bill as an 'honest but unsuccessful' attempt to solve the problem, but agreed with the *British Medical Journal* that it needed much revision. It considered that the limitations of midwife practice should be actually written into the Bill, lest midwives replaced unqualified men as assistants to medical practitioners, now that the latter's employment had been forbidden by the G.M.C. Furthermore, it was vital that the Central Board should be completely medical, and appointed by the G.M.C., and not one to which 'for some strange reason'[38] Privy Council appointees (who might even be *laymen*), had been 'imported'. The Board's rules should be entirely subject to the G.M.C., without 'interference' from the Privy Council.

The Bill was also attacked in another quarter. So far, the only criticism of proposals for midwife registration from medical women had come fourteen years before from Sophia Jex-Blake, who had condemned medical control as an infringement of midwives' rights. Now, however, there came a sudden onslaught on registration from Dr. Elizabeth Garrett Anderson, which showed that medical women, several of whom were members of the Midwives Institute,[39] were as divided on this matter as were their male colleagues. Though generally opposed to legal restrictions on women's work, on the regulation of midwives as on the regulation of prostitutes, Dr. Garrett Anderson took the popular medical line. It would be medical women, she argued, who would be the chief sufferers from the competition of the improved midwife. Worse still, an increase in the numbers of lower class women with an intimate knowledge of this branch of medicine might (through a higher criminal abortion rate) have an adverse effect on public morals.[40]

The Bill was down for debate on 11 May 1898, and in April the G.M.C. met at the Privy Council's request to consider its provisions. Also before the G.M.C. was the report of its own sub-committee appointed to watch registration. Since this sub-committee included Horsley and Brown, both members of the B.M.A.'s Midwives Bill Committee, it was not surprising that its report reflected the B.M.A. view. It accordingly condemned the proposed supervision of midwives by Medical Officers of Health, and recommended the adoption of many features of the new B.M.A. draft Bill.[41]

But while the G.M.C. as a body was not prepared to go as far as endorsing all the B.M.A.'s proposals, pressure from the anti-midwife group was strong enough so make it adopt some of the sub-committee's radical alterations. Like the B.M.A., the G.M.C. gave it as their opinion that the Bill should clearly restrict the midwife to attendance on natural labour, and require her to send for medical aid in difficult cases, thus making explicit her inferior status. Moreover, lest she should be 'inflated' into considering herself a member of a great profession, her subordinate position should be further emphasized by the replacement of State registration with annual licensing by local authorities. These licences, moreover, should not be granted without evidence of character. The possibility that the local authority might not renew her licence next year, would, it was hoped, make the midwife mind her 'P's and Q's', and, as the *Lancet* commented with satisfaction, such a restriction of independence would very much diminish the degree of official recognition of a class of persons 'who ought in the evolution of society to disappear'.[42]

A further recommendation represented a complete change of attitude on the part of the G.M.C. itself, and was in fact a great victory for the anti-midwife group. This was the proposal that practice by unqualified midwives should be banned. The G.M.C.'s change of front was hailed with glee by the *British Medical Journal* as proclaiming a 'new principle' of 'far-reaching importance' for the law of medicine as a whole, and as likely to herald G.M.C. pressure for legislation to forbid unqualified practice throughout the entire medical field.[43]

However, it had now become evident that the Government might take Private Members' time for its own business, and that after all the Bill might not be debated. Anxious to avert such an enforced delay, the Midwives Bill Committee sent a deputation to the Lord President, now the Duke of Devonshire, requesting him to make the Bill a Government measure, and to supervise its passage through Parliament. To the deputation's great disappointment, the Duke's attitude was the reverse of encouraging. Notwithstanding a petition with over 12,000 signatures for the Bill, the Duke maintained that there was 'no strong opinion' in its favour, and told the deputation that he could not advise the Government to give it their backing in face of the opposition of the medical profession. The promoters should therefore introduce a measure which would meet with 'more cordial support' from that quarter. At the same time they should come to terms with the representatives of the local authorities on whom the Bill placed the duty of local supervision but who might well not welcome the resultant financial burden.[44]

The promoters were now in a quandary. The opposition to the Bill appeared to be growing more powerful. Though the College of Physicians was still loyal, the College of Surgeons had recently pronounced against the Bill, taking the same line as the G.M.C. The G.M.C. itself had also formally expressed its disapproval, and the promoters had the task of trying to come to an agreement with that body. Yet they feared that if they accepted some of its proposals they were in danger of losing a great deal of the Parliamentary strength on which they depended in order to secure the Bill's passage into law.

In this they were right. The proposed Central Board had already been attacked by the Women's Liberal Federation for not including enough women members. Now the proposal for annual licensing came under fire from the feminist *Woman's Signal*, a journal edited by Florence Fenwick Miller, an ex-pupil of Dr. Edmunds' Ladies' Medical College. Arguing that general practitioners were often 'desperately jealous' of a clever midwife, and that the Central Board itself had a medical majority, Mrs. Miller feared that the need for the annual renewal of her licence would place the midwife's livelihood at risk from the ill-will of her professional rivals, or the calumny of gossiping neighbours. The result would be to drive educated women out of midwifery altogether. Moreover, the Lord President's request that the promoters should accede to the wishes of the G.M.C.—an all-male body—was typical of Parliament's attitude towards voteless women.[45]

There was also the thorny question of the prohibition of practice by the unqualified midwife. On this, the promoters were convinced that Parliament would persist in the Free Trade stand it had taken in the Medical and Dentists Acts. It would never interfere with the liberty of women to be attended by whom they chose, nor with that of other women to earn their living by attending them, any more than it would penalize the village blacksmith for setting bones or drawing teeth. Moreover, a ban on the unqualified woman would allow the registered midwife to assume too 'dictatorial' a position in the community, which would result in higher fees and consequent hardship for the poor whom the measure was designed to protect.[46]

Yet the solution of this problem by the public appointment of salaried midwives, as on the Continent or in Ireland, was still too radical for the Bill's supporters. Their intention was to provide the poor with midwives whose fees they could afford, not to 'pauperize' them by giving them free attendance. Still less did they wish to create a class of 'powerful and important' State employees, with a privileged position enjoyed by no other profession or trade. A further objection came from the Women's Liberal Federation, which protested at the sex discrimination inherent in the proposal to forbid practice by unqualified women while allowing unqualified men to continue as before.[47]

But these objections did not convince the opposition. If, they retorted, 1,000 mothers and 10,000 infants lost their lives annually as a result of midwives' incompetence, as the promoters claimed, Parliament would surely be willing to ban the unqualified woman. Only the year before the Legislature had confirmed the monopoly of conveyancing enjoyed by solicitors; yet there no lives were at stake. The *Lancet* was confident that after the Lord President's warning that the promoters must meet the view of the G.M.C. if they wanted Government support, Parliament would certainly 'do this service'.[48]

Taking the Lord President's advice, the promoters did indeed seek agreement with the G.M.C., and in June a delegation from the Midwives Bill Committee under Mr. Heywood Johnstone met G.M.C. representatives. To the delegates' great disappointment, the G.M.C. refused to abandon its demand for annual licensing. However, it did accept the necessity for a national list of certified midwives for the information of the local licensing authorities, but only on condition that admission to this list of itself conveyed no right to practise. On the subject of the unqualified midwife the G.M.C. was equally adamant. But although Mr. Johnstone conceded that the promoters might include a prohibitory clause in the Bill to please the G.M.C., he made it clear that this was 'wholly foreign' to their views, and that they could not undertake to defend it in Parliament.[49]

In January of the following year (1899), the sixth Midwives Bill was introduced into the Commons. In deference to G.M.C. views, the promoters had added a clause prohibiting unqualified women

from practising 'habitually and for gain', and although the Central
Board was to keep a 'Roll' of qualified midwives, annual licensing
by local authorities replaced State registration. On this last point,
the Bill did not completely meet the wishes of the G.M.C., since it
was not to be left to the local authority's discretion to grant or refuse
a licence to a midwife on the Central Board's Roll. Thus the only
purpose of annual licensing was to give the local authority information of the whereabouts of the midwives it was to supervise. However,
the G.M.C.'s insistence had secured the reinstatement of the 'good
conduct' clause which, since Bradlaugh's opposition in 1890, the
promoters had so far not dared to restore. However, women holding
the Obstetrical Society's certificate or other approved qualifications
were to be exempt from this requirement.

The promoters had also followed the Lord President's advice in
obtaining the support of the County Councils Association, which
represented the local authorities on whom the proposed local supervision would fall. But they had failed to gain the support of the
Local Government Board itself. Despite appeals to its President,
Mr. Chaplin, that he should use his influence to help carry the
measure, the department merely replied that the matter was one for
the Privy Council as the department responsible for professional
regulation.[50]

As was only to be expected, some educated midwives felt betrayed
by the action of the Midwives Bill Committee (on which the Midwives' Institute had been represented), in jettisoning State registration, and, as they saw it, handing over midwives' interests to a rival
profession, in obedience to the 'decrees' of the G.M.C.[51] Some of
these women were allies of Mrs. Bedford Fenwick, and had hoped
for State registration along with the trained nurse, rather than with
the midwife of only three months' training—or none at all. To them
the new Bill was a graver threat than any of its predecessors. If it
passed into law there would be no State registration—of any sort—
for midwives. Instead, *every* midwife, however well educated and
trained, would be subjected willy-nilly to licensing by the local
authority on the same level as cab-drivers and stall-holders.

One of Mrs. Fenwick's leading supporters, Miss Margaret Breay,
herself a midwife and ex-matron, expressed her indignation in the
Nursing Record. The Bill's obvious purpose, she protested, was not to
mend midwives, but to *end* them. Why, then, had the journal of the
Midwives' Institute, *Nursing Notes*, made no comment on the
'seriousness' of the situation? Miss Breay doubted the promoters'
assurances that the midwife's licence would be renewed automatically each year, fearing that it would often be arbitrarily withheld on
the evidence of the midwife's medical competitors. She also ques-

tioned how fair a hearing a midwife would receive at the hands of a Central Board consisting almost entirely of medical men. No educated woman, she predicted, would come forward to work under the Bill's 'humiliating' conditions—the joint product of the professional antagonism of doctors and the vindictive determination of less broad-minded men to 'prevent at all costs, and by any means, the organisation of women'.[52]

These criticisms were quickly endorsed by another *Record* correspondent. The plain truth, wrote 'Lancashire Midwife', was that the medical profession was determined not to allow either midwives or nurses to be registered by the State. Midwives had been 'sacrificed' by the Midwives Bill Committee, and trained nurses 'sold into bondage' by the Royal British Nurses' Association. This neglect of their interest by bodies expressly formed to secure their professional status was convincing proof that no matters affecting women's work should be entrusted to men.[53]

The opinion of 'Lancashire Midwife' was representative of a new local group of militant midwives. This was the 'Manchester Midwives' Society', founded two years before with a membership of sixty certificated midwives from Manchester and surrounding areas. The Society was in fact direct heir to Maria Firth's Association of 1872, and, unlike the Midwives' Institute, objected strongly to any form of registration under medical control. The interests of medical men, the Society believed, were contrary to those of midwives, and while better training for midwives was necessary, registration of this sort was not. It had therefore opposed the 1898 Bill.[54]

It is not surprising that 'Lancashire Midwife' felt so strongly. The Obstetrical Society's view had always been that the registered midwife should only attend the poor, a view recently expounded with great conviction by Dr. W. Alexander, Visiting Surgeon at the Liverpool Workhouse Infirmary. According to Alexander, midwives were suitable for poor women, who, being stronger, had less need of skilled assistance. Moreover, registration would have the merit of putting midwives in their proper place—doing the hard, tedious, ill-paid work appropriate for women. 'By training and control', explained Dr. Alexander,

women will have their fair and natural share of, and emoluments from, midwifery work, whilst medical men will occupy a more manly and dignified position in regard to labours amongst the poor than by the drudgery necessitated by personally attending badly paid confinements, where the wear-and-tear, anxiety, and exposure lead to premature old age, and where the necessity of quickly terminating a case sometimes leads to dangerous or fatal measures being adopted, that the patience and leisure of the midwife would avoid.[55]

The B.M.A., in the meantime, had prepared even more stringent proposals for the control of midwives. Duties of licensing and supervision they now wished to see laid on a committee of three medical practitioners (not teachers or examiners of midwives) appointed by the local authority, rather than on the Medical Officer of Health, who, they maintained, would be either too busy, or not sufficiently independent. Moreover, there should be no exemption for women with the Obstetrical Society's certificate from the requirement that existing midwives should produce evidence of good character before being admitted to the Roll. Taken together these two proposals ensured that even the educated lady midwives of the Midwives' Institute would have to seek their licences on the same footing as the lowest Gamp at the hands of a committee of general practitioners who might well be their rivals for practice. Further, lying-in homes run by midwives (but not, however, those run by medical men) should be subject to local authority inspection.[56]

As before, the Central Midwives Board was to be an all-medical body drawn from different districts of the country, from which teachers and examiners of midwives should be excluded. In its claim that such a constitution would make the Board more 'representative', the B.M.A. was anxious only for representation of the general practitioner, whom it wished to see assume a dominating position in the registration machinery at both central and local level. It was not at all concerned with the representation of those whose livelihood the Board might control. While conceding that the Midwives' Institute possibly knew more about midwives than other organizations represented on the Board, the B.M.A.'s sub-committee on the Bill considered that for the Institute itself to be represented would be a 'departure from ordinary procedure'.[57]

The promoters' Bill came up for debate unexpectedly on 12 April 1899. The attack on the Bill was led by a new recruit to the opposition, the popular journalist T. P. O'Connor, one of the Liverpool members. Apart from this, the time available was very short, and it was inevitable that the Bill should be talked out. Its supporters were thus faced with the task of keeping up the momentum of the campaign until the Bill could be brought in again the following year. Accordingly, the Association for the Registration of Midwives sought to allay the fears of those of its supporters who had been alarmed by the Bill's stringent new provisions. Defending annual licensing, the Association urged the necessity of keeping track of individual midwives if poor mothers were to be protected from the Gamps, and confessed itself 'baffled' by the 'strongly expressed opinions' of 'one or two lady-writers' who were well-aware of the evils which annual licensing was designed to prevent.[58]

These 'strongly expressed opinions' were, as was to be expected, warmly endorsed by Mrs. Bedford Fenwick, who accused the Midwives' Institute of 'sacrificing midwives' interests' by supporting the Bill. The separate registration of midwives she still regarded as 'a dangerous precedent', complaining that both the medical opposition to nurse registration, and the promoters of the Midwives Bill, were 'compromising the situation', instead of adopting a 'bold statesmanlike policy' for the joint registration of midwives and trained nurses.[59]

The arrival on the scene of the Manchester Midwives' Society had not made things any easier for the Midwives' Institute, which was now supporting a Bill far less favourable to midwives than the 1898 version. The Institute acknowledged that the new Bill was 'inferior', but held that the need for regulation in the interests of poor mothers was so great that, provided certain clauses safeguarding midwives' rights were retained, any Bill was better than nothing.[60] Conscious of the weak position midwives were in, it warned the Manchester Society that if midwives insisted on opposing every Bill not framed exactly according to their wishes some Bill 'much more detrimental' to their interests would be introduced and might well pass.[61]

The Institute had also to suffer the embarrassment of being confused with the Manchester Society itself, which, ignoring the Institute's warning, had petitioned the Commons against the Bill. Some supporters of registration had been alarmed by the Manchester association's aspirations to be considered a learned society, and its demands for professional independence for midwives.[62] The new Society had thus provided the Institute's opponents with extra ammunition, which they hastened to use. To make matters worse for the Institute, early in 1900 there appeared in certain newspapers an anonymous advertisement advocating support for the Bill, which, it urged, would 'practically abolish man-midwifery'. Despite a disclaimer by the Institute, the advertisement was seized on by the opposition as further evidence of a feminist bid to regain the whole field of midwifery for women.[63]

Early in the year the new Bill was published. Though in most respects it followed the 1899 Bill, it introduced an important new feature. This provided a solution to the problem—pointed out by John Simon over twenty years before—of financing the central regulation machinery if midwives proved too poor to bear the necessary cost through examination and registration fees. The medical men among the Bill's promoters had at last recognized the force of Simon's argument that registration could not function without financial support from local government. Accordingly, the new clause proposed to lay on County Councils, in proportion to the number of midwives practising in their respective areas, the burden of any deficit which the Central Midwives Board might annually face, thus departing from the usual practice of requiring members of a profession to meet the whole cost of their registration machinery. In recognition of this new liability a representative of the County Councils' Association was to have a seat on the Board.

The *Lancet*, which had taken a fairly non-committal line when the Bill was published the year before, now decided to test medical opinion on the issue. This it attempted to do by means of a questionnaire sent to the 20,000 or so members of the profession on the English Register. Of the third who replied, a fifth said they favoured the Bill, a tenth were indifferent, while the rest opposed it. From these results the *Lancet* concluded (unjustifiably, considering the large number who had not replied) that four-fifths of the profession were against the Bill, on the grounds that it 'infringed the Medical Acts'. Pressure should therefore be put on the promoters to meet the profession's requirements.[64]

As usual, the B.M.A. had made arrangements for blocking the Bill. But on 9 March its supporters in the Commons took advantage of an unexpected opportunity to bring it up for its second reading, and it was consequently debated before a small House. Like the previous year's Bill, it was vehemently opposed by T. P. O'Connor. The promoters' 'philanthropic feeling', O'Connor claimed, had induced them to overstate the incompetence of the untrained midwife. Furthermore, official recognition of midwives would give them an exaggerated sense of their skill, and lead to an increase in malpractice and abortion. O'Connor was supported by two Irish medical M.P.s, Drs. Ambrose and Tanner, though as before the Bill did not apply to Ireland. Despite their arguments, and despite the absence of its leading supporters, the Bill passed after a short debate with 4–1 majority.[65] The Commons had thus approved in principle the regulation of midwife practice, as the Lords had done in 1895.

The Bill's success caused consternation among its opponents. Dr. Rentoul, stirred to renewed activity by this development, appealed for redoubled effort. In view of the 'emergency', a special meeting of the B.M.A. Council was called, and the *British Medical Journal* urged medical men to write to their M.P.s, especially to those on the Standing Committee on Law to which the Bill had been referred. Indeed, several M.P.s on the Committee were well disposed to the opposition—including Lloyd George, who put on record his support for George Brown in the fight against 'this rotten Bill'. But although these members attempted to amend the Bill to meet the B.M.A.'s wishes, they were unsuccessful, and it passed on to await its report stage virtually unaltered.[66]

Even facing defeat the opposition remained divided. Brown's *General Practitioner* (the Medical Practitioners' Association's new journal) and Dr. Bedford Fenwick's *Medical Times*, both lashed the B.M.A. for producing a Bill of its own and not opposing all midwife legislation. The B.M.A., fulminated the *General Practitioner*, was nothing more than 'a broken reed' to which it was useless to entrust the interests of the profession in medico-political matters. The *Medical Times* warned that the 'fatal results' of allowing chemists to be registered outside the control of the medical profession would be repeated in the case of midwives. Moreover, the Bill would be a precedent for the registration of nurses, also independent of medical control. As usual, the journal supported the *Nursing Record* in calling for a Select Committee on the joint registration of midwives and nurses.[67]

Commenting on the situation, the independent *Practitioner* warned members of the anti-midwife party of where their actions were leading. They might blame their defeat on the B.M.A., the G.M.C., and the Obstetrical Society, as well as on 'drawing-room philanthropists and Machiavellian midwives', but it was their own 'shop-counter attitude' which had most damaged their cause. Impatient of their outpourings, the journal appealed to the *Lancet* and the *British Medical Journal* to apply 'the closure' to these 'scribblers and stump-orators' who, although of no account in the profession, had put themselves forward as its champions, disgusting all reasonable men with their agitation for monopoly. The poor response to the *Lancet*'s questionnaire showed clearly enough that a large part of the profession did not care whether the Bill passed or not.[68]

But there was still time to secure the amendment of the Bill, and both the G.M.C. and the B.M.A. sought to enlist Government support for their objections. The G.M.C. requested that the Privy Council should allow the inclusion of a clause restricting the midwife to attendance on natural labour, while the B.M.A. approached the Solicitor-General on this and its other proposals. Neither of these approaches was successful. The Privy Council was adamant that the limitation of the midwife's practice would be best dealt with in the rules of the Central Midwives Board, which in any case must be submitted to the G.M.C. for its approval, a position which, despite vigorous opposition from Horsley and Brown, the great majority of the G.M.C. agreed to accept.[69] The Bill thus received the G.M.C.'s general approval, to the great disgust of the B.M.A. and the Medical Practitioners' Association, both of whom condemned the G.M.C.

M.M.—6

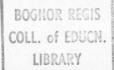

for abandoning the profession's case. Without such a penal clause, complained the *British Medical Journal*, a midwife who had not sent for the doctor in a case of abnormal labour could only be punished by the remote Central Board, rather than in the local courts, with consequent local publicity.[70]

The Bill came on for its report stage late on 27 June, when there were only fifty minutes left. Predictably, it was opposed by Sir Walter Foster, putting the B.M.A. view, and also by lay M.P.s who looked back with regret to the 'good old time' before the modern craze for examination and registration. There was even more serious opposition, however. At the last moment, the Home Office had come out against the Bill. As the department responsible for law enforcement, it had already been consulted several times by Mr. Johnstone in the course of framing the Bill, and interviews with its officials had resulted in agreement. It was thus a complete surprise when at two days' notice the department produced no less than sixty-nine amendments, threatening to oppose the Bill if they were not accepted. Since these included an abandonment of the clauses on annual licensing and the prohibition of unqualified practice, both questions of principle on which Mr. Johnstone had given an undertaking to the G.M.C., he could not move them himself without risking the charge of a breach of faith. Neither could he risk the overt opposition of the Home Office. In consequence, to the great mystification of his opponents, he talked the Bill out.

The change of front on the part of the Home Office was not made public at this stage. It appears to have originated with the department's political heads, Charles Ritchie, the Home Secretary, and Jesse Collings, the Under Secretary, who, significantly, had voted against the Bill's second reading. However, it was only after the Bill had passed its Committee stage that Ritchie had made known his views that several of its most important clauses must be amended. Ritchie's objection was that the Bill's proposals went far beyond, or were contrary to, the recommendations of the 1893 Select Committee. In particular, he condemned the prohibition of unqualified practice, 'strongly deprecating' the 'unnecessary multiplication' of small criminal offences. Such a ban, he considered, would create a monopoly for the registered midwife, and cause hardship to poor mothers by preventing them from having the attendant of their choice. Annual licensing, he contended, would be 'cumbrous, vexatious, and capable of oppressive use'; a system of annual notification as operated in the case of foster mothers under the amended Infant Life Protection legislation would be quite sufficient. Ritchie was also hostile to the clause which gave the G.M.C. a vote over the rules to be made by the Central Midwives Board for the control and limitation of midwife practice. This concession to the G.M.C., he pointed out, was contrary to the recommendations of the Select Committee, which had proposed that the final say on the rules should rest with the Privy Council. Moreover, it was wrong to give a 'private body' like the G.M.C. so much power over other members of the public. Since there would in any case be a medical majority on the Midwives Board, to allow the G.M.C. control over its rules would be to place the whole execution of the Act in the hands of the medical profession. Yet it could not be forgotten that there was 'a great deal of jealousy' on the part of a large body of practitioners over the midwife question; in these circumstances the G.M.C.'s power over the rules should be carefully limited, and made subject to the approval of a Government department as 'an independent and disinterested body'.[71]

None of this appears to have been generally known, however, and despite the failure of the Bill, the Association for Promoting the Registration of Midwives was well pleased with the situation. Although, because of lack of private members' time at the end of the session, the Bill could not be further proceeded with that year, the fact that it had reached the report stage was considered to represent 'tremendous progress'. This time there had been considerable parliamentary support for the Bill, and the Association was able to report that M.P.s no longer minded talking about midwives, in private or public, and that the opposition's will to oppose was becoming weaker.[72] Support in the country at large continued to grow, and the Association now had the active co-operation of the radical liberal reform group the Fabian Society, and of C. S. Loch, influential Secretary of the Charity Organization Society. A deputation to the Lord President in June had found him 'much more encouraging' than two years before, promising to bring the matter seriously before his Government colleagues, and offering the services of his department to help draft the Bill. However, he had still made it clear that he did not contemplate making it a Government measure.[73]

The outlook was thus reasonably hopeful for the following year. The Association for Promoting the Registration of Midwives, whose well-to-do philanthropic leadership advocated regulation primarily in order to protect poor mothers and their infants, rather than to elevate the status of midwives, might well congratulate themselves that the long struggle must soon end in success. Not surprisingly, their satisfaction was not generally shared by the defenders of women's rights, the *Englishwoman's Review* in particular condemning the Bill's 'insulting' provision for local licensing.[74] Nor did the Bill please those educated midwives who, while accepting an element of medical control, still looked forward to recognized professional status through State registration. For them, as for the most militant of anti-midwife general practitioners, the enactment of the Bill would spell defeat.

The anti-midwife party, however, had also achieved considerable success, despite its protests that the Bill allowed the midwife *too much* independence. It was through its efforts that the promoters had been forced to accept proposals subjecting midwives to a greater degree of medical control than most of them had wished. Though not as restrictive as some of the midwife regulation schemes instituted over the past decade in certain parts of the United States, a measure on these lines would represent victory for those medical men who, like many of their American counterparts, viewed regulation merely as a short-term instrument to control the midwife until they themselves could supersede her.[75] This development, it was confidently expected, could not be far distant. In the more affluent and educated world of the future, every woman would be delivered by a doctor, and the midwife, a relic of a less civilized past, would vanish from the scene.[76]

CHAPTER EIGHT

The Midwives Act, 1902

The progress which the Midwives Bill had made in 1900 meant that its successor would be introduced at the earliest opportunity. Since the formation seven years previously of the two associations campaigning for registration, the movement had gained much influential public support. In addition, the number of women seeking the Obstetrical Society's certificate—many in anticipation of registration—had more than doubled, and in 1900 reached over 900, of whom 754 were successful. Yet the promoters were as dependent as before on their luck in the Private Members' ballot for the introduction of their Bill into the Commons, and their lack of success in 1901 meant that it could not be brought in at all that year.

Nonetheless, the controversy over registration raged unabated in the *British Medical Journal*. In the main the arguments were the same as those brought forward when the first Midwives Bill was introduced in 1890. The real object of the registration party, protested its opponents, was to provide an occupation for the increasing numbers of women in the population, if not to oust men from midwifery altogether. Registration would create an inferior order of medical practitioners; there was no more need to 'legalize' midwives than herbalists, bone-setters, aurists, opticians, curers of hernia or venereal disease, 'restorers of manly function', or other 'irregular practitioners'. Midwives were quite unnecessary, since the services of a doctor could be provided through provident clubs and dispensaries, lying-in charities, and the Poor Law Medical Service.[1]

However, probably because of the changed social climate resulting from the defeats of the Boer War, there was this time more support for the idea that medical attendance on poor childbearing women should be financed from the public purse. Significantly, it was increasingly argued that such provision should be made not by the Guardians but by the local health authority, on the grounds that this was a matter of the public health rather than the relief of destitution. Indeed, one leading anti-registrationist went so far as to propound the revolutionary doctrine that it was the duty of the State in its own interests to provide this service, as it did in the case of vaccination and education, free to all, irrespective of income.

Advocates of registration, as before, challenged the assumption held by many members of the anti-midwife camp that all 'respectable' working-class women could afford the doctor's guinea, and a medical woman, Dr. Gerda Jacobi, reminded the profession of the extensive poverty uncovered by Charles Booth's monumental survey of London life and labour. But even the poorest women, Dr. Jacobi insisted, would not consent to be 'bundled into the workhouse' at the sweet will of the medical profession, merely in order to be attended by a doctor. Furthermore, a study of the principles of political economy would soon reveal the impracticability of the proposed extension of free services.

But there were other considerations besides financial ones. Many women, Dr. Jacobi claimed, would not agree to being attended by a man. Another supporter of registration, a Dr. Farrar, agreed, defending the right of women to the free choice of attendant. Though the better-off might prefer a medical man because he could administer chloroform, it would be 'utterly preposterous' to demand that a natural process should never take place without a doctor present.

Nor, as Dr. F. R. Humphreys, Secretary of the Midwives' Registration Association, patiently reminded the profession, was a Midwives Act necessary to make midwifery an occupation for women, or to protect midwives' interests. Midwives existed already, and were free to practise as and where they pleased under the protection of the common law. Medical men, who were under the supervision of the G.M.C., were more restricted in their practice than midwives. Although it was essential that the Act should place proper limitations on the practice of midwives, it was certain that Parliament would never place them 'unreservedly' in the hands of the medical profession.

This year (1901) was also the year for the election of the profession's direct representatives to the G.M.C., and as in 1891 and 1896, the dominating issue was midwives' registration. Two of the existing representatives, Dr. Glover and Mr. George Brown, were standing again for the two seats vacant for England and Wales. Dr. George Jackson of Plymouth (like Brown, a candidate of the militant Medical Practitioners' Association) and Dr. Samuel Woodcock, a general practitioner and member of the B.M.A. Parliamentary Bills Committee, who had shared in the framing of the B.M.A.'s own very stringent Bill, were the other serious candidates.

As before, Dr. Glover advocated registration. He pointed out, however, that he had nevertheless opposed the 1900 Bill as not stringent enough in the control it would exercise over the registered midwife. The aim of legislation should be to provide safe midwives for the poor, but for the poor only. For this reason he would resist any move to make midwives 'highly trained women', indeed, he looked forward to the time when *every* woman would be delivered by a registered medical practitioner. Midwives were necessary for the time being, however, and those who were against legislation of any kind should realize that the Government would never support them. A Midwives Act was inevitable; the profession should therefore take care not to lose the chance of shaping it according to its wishes.

Unmoved by this plea, Brown and Jackson reiterated their out-and-out opposition to legislation, while Dr. Woodcock took the same line as Dr. Glover. All four candidates agreed that the local health authority should pay the fee for those women who wished to be attended by a doctor but who were too poor to pay him themselves. They were also unanimous in advocating the amendment of the Medical Acts to allow the suppression of unqualified medical practice—a decision of great significance for any Midwives Bill.

So far discussion of the 'midwife question' had been confined almost entirely to the medical journals. Now, in the autumn of 1901, two childbirth fatalities occurred which were to bring the question to general notice. There was, of course, nothing unusual in the fact that two women had died in childbirth, or that they had died for want of skilled attention. But their deaths had highlighted the problems which might face the midwife, when, as would almost certainly be required under the provisions of any Midwives Act, she called in the doctor to a difficult labour. At the same time the behaviour of the doctors concerned in these two cases had done much to discredit medical opposition to registration. In the first case, in Swanscombe, Kent, the husband had applied to three doctors in succession, offering them half the guinea fee on the spot, and promising the rest later. All three had refused, having earlier agreed among themselves not to 'follow' midwives. In a similar case in Stepney, in consequence of which the elderly incompetent midwife was imprisoned for manslaughter, the doctor called by the husband had excused himself on the (unjustified) plea that if he attended, the G.M.C. could charge him with 'covering' an unqualified practitioner.

The Swanscombe case gave rise to a lively correspondence in the *British Medical Journal*. Two correspondents condemned the action of the Swanscombe doctors. Several, however, defended it, arguing that doctors must protect themselves, not only from too much unpaid

attendance, but also from the danger that they would be blamed
for deaths caused by the incompetence of the midwife. Others were
prepared to go even further. To provide medical attendance for his
family, wrote one hard-liner, was 'just as much' the duty of the poor
man as it was for the rich. No-one could seriously believe that there
were 'respectable' women who were unable to afford the 'ordinary'
fee of 10s. to 21s.; the whole problem generally arose from 'want of
thrift' on the part of either husband or wife. The Swanscombe case
was 'a good wholesome lesson' to teach the poor that they could not
'shirk their responsibilities', and the profession should be grateful to
the Swanscombe doctors for their stand.

Those medical men who felt that some reform was needed proposed different lines of action. Some agreed with Dr. Glover's
proposal that local health authorities should be empowered to pay
the fee of doctors called in to emergencies. Others thought that such
cases could safely be referred to the Poor Law. But, as pointed out
by the *British Medical Journal* and several correspondents, many
Guardians would not sanction payment to their Medical Officer in
cases where the family had not first obtained a Midwifery Order
from the Relieving Officer.

Midwives, however, and their lay supporters, attacked such
collectivist solutions as likely to undermine the independence of the
poor. It was their experience that many women preferred to work
and scrape and pay the midwife themselves, rather than seek free
attendance by applying to a hospital subscriber for a 'hospital letter'
or to the Receiving Officer for a Poor Law Order. There was also the
advantage that the midwife, besides attending the birth, would
generally act as a nurse as well. This independent spirit should not
be sapped by any scheme for free medical aid; the fact that the
Swanscombe husband had offered the doctors half their fee proved
that he was not a case for parish relief.[2]

The concerted action of the Swanscombe doctors gave great
satisfaction to the anti-midwife interests. However, when pressed by
the medical supporters of registration to declare his attitude on the
Swanscombe doctors' behaviour, the G.M.C. candidate Brown had
preferred not to commit himself. Other medical men were more
outspoken, however. If all doctors refused to follow midwives, wrote
one *British Medical Journal* correspondent, this would be the end of the
midwife question once and for all. Dr. McCook Weir, who nine years
before had refused to answer the call of a nursing association midwife,
welcomed the Swanscombe doctors' stand as proving that the 'mere
male' was still master of the situation. Medical men, he urged,
should drop their 'sham philanthropy', and unite for the common
good of the profession.

The example of the Swanscombe doctors was clearly being followed elsewhere. In some areas it was so successful that trained midwives working in private practice or for maternity charities were having to leave the district rather than take responsibility for abnormal cases on their own. As Miss Rosalind Paget, Treasurer of the Midwives' Institute, complained to *The Times*, this development might well have the effect of driving out the trained midwife altogether, leaving all midwife practice to unqualified women.[3]

The Swanscombe case had now become a *cause célèbre*, and the subsequent correspondence in the *British Medical Journal* in support of the Swanscombe doctors furnished registrationists with a golden opportunity to discredit the opposition, and during December several letters advocating registration appeared in *The Times*. By the end of the month, the *British Medical Journal*, greatly alarmed at the adverse publicity the profession was receiving, warned medical men against any 'systematic refusal' to 'follow' midwives. The Swanscombe and Stepney cases, it pointed out, had already given the promoters of the Midwives Bill additional ammunition for their cause, and when the next Bill was introduced in the New Year it would have the backing of many influential people, including M.P.s, and there would be little hope of amending it in the House.

In the meantime, the election of the direct representatives to the G.M.C. had taken place. Shortly before the election Dr. Glover had withdrawn because of illness, and the result was a sweeping victory for the anti-registrationist candidates, Jackson and Brown. This was the vote for the extremists which the *British Medical Journal* had feared, and which in the opinion of the *Hospital* signified that the B.M.A. could no longer claim to speak for the profession. Although only 43% of those on the Medical Register had voted, the *Hospital* was right in pointing out that any unanimous move on the part of the profession to put forward the B.M.A. Bill as an alternative to the promoters' Bill was now knocked on the head. Those who had supported the 'impossible programme' of Jackson and Brown had probably actually contributed to the ultimate success of the very Bill to which they were so strongly opposed.[4]

In the New Year the promoters were lucky in the Private Members' ballot, and the Bill was put down to be debated on 26 February. This gave the promoters an advantage they had not enjoyed on earlier occasions, and, as the *British Medical Journal* warned its readers, the large number of petitions in favour of registration, together with the fact that the promoters had friends in the Cabinet,[5] gave it a good chance of passing its second reading.

Despite its warning to the extremists, it had never occurred to the *British Medical Journal* that the B.M.A. itself might have been too extreme in its opposition to the 1900 Bill for the success of its cause. The B.M.A.'s own draft Bill proposed to put midwives, whose interests were to be entirely unrepresented, largely under the control of general practitioners at both central and local level. Now the Swanscombe case had shown how dangerous for midwives this could be. Although the G.M.C. had finally approved the 1900 Bill, the B.M.A. still hoped to gain further concessions when it was reintroduced into Parliament. Confident in the knowledge that four years previously the Lord President had told the promoters that they had no hope of Government support unless they came to terms with the G.M.C., the opposition had never envisaged the possibility that one day the promoters might be strong enough to ignore this agreement and draft the Bill they really wanted.

Yet this is precisely what had happened, and when the Bill was published, its provisions came as a great shock to the B.M.A. Far from being a more stringent version of its predecessor, it had reverted to the form and spirit of the Bill of 1898. Although the word 'registration' did not appear in the title, and 'Roll' was used instead of 'Register', the Bill returned to State registration, substituting for the annual licensing of the 1900 Bill the simple requirement that midwives intending to practise in a certain county should annually notify their intention to the local authority. Further, the clause prohibiting unqualified practice had been cut out, leaving only the protection of the title of 'midwife'.

The amendments to the 1900 Bill were the result of the intervention of the Home Office at the report stage of that Bill. At this point the promoters had been forced to weigh the value of their 1898 undertaking to the G.M.C. against the certain death of the Bill if Home Office opposition were to continue. Influenced by the fact that their concessions to the G.M.C. had still not brought them its support, they had decided to adopt the Home Office position on these clauses, which in any case accorded with their own views.[6] Discussions with the Home Office, Local Government Board and Privy Council Office followed, as a result of which the sanction of these departments was secured for their proposals.[7] With Government approval, and increasing public and Parliamentary support, they were now strong enough to defy the G.M.C.

But the promoters had gone even further than a mere repudiation of their 1898 undertaking to the G.M.C. The 1902 Bill, in contrast to all its predecessors, proposed that the Central Midwives Board should be completely independent of the G.M.C. During the Committee stage of the 1900 Bill an amendment to this effect had been proposed by Mr. Atherley Jones, M.P. Mr. Jones had told members of letters he had received from medical opponents of registration who expected the G.M.C. to make the Board's rules so strict as to discourage midwives from practice. On that occasion, however, Mr. Jones' amendment had been resisted by the promoters, who were anxious to keep faith with the G.M.C.[8]

Since then the Home Office had informed the promoters of its opposition on this point, as on others. In the eyes of the Liberal-Unionist Parliamentary Under-Secretary, Jesse Collings, the G.M.C. was 'the most exclusive and over-bearing Trades Union in the country',[9] and Collings accordingly refused to allow complete power over the Board's rules to rest in its hands. In the new Bill it was to be the Privy Council, not the G.M.C., which was to undertake the formation of the Central Board and to have the final say on its rules.

Immediately the Bill was published it was bitterly attacked in the medical press as the 'worst' yet. Dr. Fenwick's *Medical Times* reiterated its call for a Select Committee to consider legislation for nurses and midwives together. The *Lancet* denounced the Bill as 'a distinct blow' to medical men, promising as it did to 'semi-educated women' many of the privileges enjoyed by the medical profession, by contrast, 'a highly educated body, with a strict professional code and a recognised social position'. On the same tack, the *British Medical Journal* protested that registration would create a superior midwife who would rob the medical man of his better-off patients while it did nothing to protect the poor from the Gamps. It had always been the promoters' intention to establish an independent order of practitioners and for all the good such an Act would do Parliament might just as well 'legalize' herbalists and bone-setters. Again, it was 'extraordinary' that the Home Office had advised the promoters to drop the clause prohibiting unqualified practice in order to follow the precedent of the Medical Acts when it well knew these to be greatly in need of amendment in the same direction.

Both journals regretted the disappearance of the clause requiring midwives to take out annual licences, since annual licensing would have prevented the registered midwife from appearing as an independent practitioner in the eyes of the public. The new independence proposed for the Central Midwives Board, complained the *British Medical Journal*, would make it the 'exact counterpart' of the G.M.C., thus misleading the public and infringing the Medical Acts. The whole machinery of registration had been taken out of the hands of the medical profession, and even medical men who favoured legislation could not support the Bill in this form. All the influence the profession could command should be brought to bear on Parliament to secure its rejection.

But the time for the opposition to rally was short. This time the promoters had been lucky with the ballot, and the Bill was down for its second reading as early as 26 February, only a few days after its publication. In consequence, the medical weeklies had been allowed only one opportunity to comment before the debate. The G.M.C., which happened to be in special session to consider a dispute with the Royal College of Surgeons, was able to make time to discuss the Bill two days before it came before the House. Complaining that its provisions were 'at variance' with the principles it had previously adopted, the Council informed the Lord President that in its view the Bill ought not to pass 'in its present form', while individual members expressed their anger at the promoters' 'broken faith'.

It is an ill wind, however, that blows nobody any good, and Mrs. Bedford Fenwick was quick to detect the good in the changed circumstances for her cherished project of a Nurses' Registration Act. In spite of her repeated attempts to get the registration of nurses considered together with that of midwives, the latest of which had been an approach by the Matrons' Council, a group of hospital matrons favouring nurse registration, to the G.M.C. in January, she had failed. Now, as a result of the great growth in support for the Midwives Bill, it was clear that her project was out of the question. If the promoters were strong enough to ignore the wishes of the G.M.C., there was obviously no advantage to be gained for nurses by opposing the Bill. So, after twelve years' bitter and unrelenting opposition to midwife registration, Mrs. Fenwick found no difficulty in adjusting to the new situation. Abandoning her alliance with her husband's *Medical Times*—still frantically trying to organize opposition to the Bill—she herself prepared gracefully to accept a Midwives Act as a precedent for nurse registration.

Mrs. Fenwick also welcomed the disappearance of the clause requiring midwives to take out annual licences like 'hawkers and publicans', pointing out, justifiably, that alone among the nursing journals the *Nursing Record* had consistently protested against this 'objectionable provision'. Indeed, in taking this position the *Record* had reflected the views of many midwives more accurately than the London-based Midwives' Institute and the well-to-do leadership of the Association for the Registration of Midwives. Thanking the journal for its consistent defence of women's liberties, a Manchester midwife regretted that 'London midwives, or their representatives, and ladies who don't know what it is to earn a living' had ever tolerated these 'medical suggestions'.[10]

The removal of the Central Midwives Board from the jurisdiction of the G.M.C. received Mrs. Fenwick's whole-hearted approval. Since her break with the medical leadership of the Royal British Nurses Association, Mrs. Fenwick was no longer as keen as she had been on a large element of medical control in the professional organization of nurses or midwives. Her revised view was that medical men should appear only as consultants on the regulating bodies of these professions, and, like other campaigners for women's rights, she regretted that midwives themselves were not to constitute the majority of members on the Midwives Board.

On 26 February the debate on the Bill opened in a crowded House, and with a general sentiment in its favour. This was in striking contrast to previous occasions, when promoters had sought in vain to interest the great body of M.P.s in the subject. The change was due to two factors. One was the hard work put in by the promoters to gain Parliamentary support. The other was the new political climate—the result of the Boer War, in which a small nation of farmers had for a considerable period defied the might of the British Empire. The fear that the race was deteriorating physically, together with increasing concern over the falling birth-rate, led many to question Britain's ability to play the imperial role which she had set herself, or even to defend her own shores against the growing power of Germany. Against this background of uncertainty and the new search for 'National Efficiency' the children of the poor again came to be spoken of as the physical capital of the nation. Pleas for safe attendance on poor childbearing women were thus more likely to gain a sympathetic hearing.

The Bill was introduced by Lord Cecil Manners, a young unmarried man. This in itself was an indication of the general change in attitude which had taken place in the twelve years since 1890, when discussion of the midwife question was considered either a 'huge joke', or 'not quite proper', and the Bill itself had occasioned much ribald merriment in the House.[11] It was a measure of the support which registration had gained that Mr. T. P. O'Connor, who had strenuously opposed the more stringent 1900 Bill, now claimed to be no more than a 'vigilant critic' of this one. Though medical M.P.s opposing the Bill included Sir John Tuke, a member of the G.M.C., and Sir Walter Foster, the promoters enjoyed the support of two medical men who carried more weight in the House— Dr. Farquharson, also a leading figure in the B.M.A., and Sir Michael Foster, member for London University.

Lord Cecil Manners made the general case for the Bill,[12] deploring the fact that Britain was alone among the civilized countries of Europe in having no system of midwife regulation. But the speech of his seconder, Mr. de Tatton Egerton, Chairman of the General Lying-in Hospital, was more noteworthy in that it showed how far some of the Bill's promoters were prepared to go in publicly expressing their antagonism to the G.M.C. Attacking that body for its 'dog-in-the-manger' attitude on midwife legislation, Mr. Egerton recalled how it had consistently refused to undertake the task of registration itself, yet had opposed every Bill brought forward by others.

Sir John Tuke moved the Bill's rejection on behalf of the G.M.C. Concentrating on the lack of a clause banning the unqualified midwife, he protested that this omission 'eviscerated' the measure, which, while placing the registered midwife under tight restriction, left the ignorant, incompetent woman to practise how she pleased. Despite the Home Office claim that such a clause would create a new class of offence, Sir John Tuke pointed out that there was pre-cedent for such prohibition in the Apothecaries Act of 1815—still enforced—and also in the law governing the practice of solicitors.

Other opposition speakers paraded the old arguments that registration would encourage the midwife to usurp the doctor's role, would result in an increase in criminal abortions, and would contravene the 1886 Medical Act. The G.M.C., Sir Walter Foster reminded the House, had recently forbidden registered practitioners to employ unqualified men, however experienced, as their assistants. Yet the Midwives Bill proposed to give legal recognition to a class of women with very short training, whom medical men might then freely employ. In any case, a register of trained women would be useless without the prohibition of unqualified practice. It might be nailed on the church door, but the poor would always send for the woman who was popular locally, trained or not. If the public were really to be protected, the unqualified woman should be banned and all midwives made to take out annual licences, in order that they might be kept 'respectable' and prevented from practising as abortionists.

The opposition also condemned the proposal to put the Midwives Board under the Privy Council rather than the G.M.C. The G.M.C., Sir Walter complained, had been 'practically struck out' of the Bill, and the regulation machinery thus deprived of 'central medical control'. The fact that the Midwives Board was to have a majority of medical members was not enough, since these were only to be responsible to the Privy Council. Worse still, one of them was to represent the Midwives' Institute, 'a nameless, if not imaginary body', 'unknown' to the medical profession, whereas 'that splendid institution, the Royal Nurses' Association', was not to be repre-sented. This eulogy of the R.B.N.A. however, was merely an opposi-tion ploy to persuade M.P.s that the midwife question was only part of the larger issue of nurse registration. Warning the House that directly the Midwives Bill became law it would be followed by a Nurses Bill, Sir Walter called on the Home Secretary to refer both matters to a Select Committee.

None of this made much impression, however. Mr. Eugene Wason, M.P. for Clackmannan and Kinross, thought that the promoters were to be congratulated on obtaining the Government's sanction for their proposals, even at the expense of agreement with the G.M.C. The abandonment of annual licensing was defended by Mr. Heywood Johnstone on the grounds that many midwives had objected to being put on the same 'low plane' as applicants for dog and gun licences. Annual notification, on the other hand, was more convenient, and would serve the same purpose. The opposition's proposal to prohibit the unqualified midwife was dismissed by Dr. Farquharson as a 'hopeless Utopian dream', while Mr. Johnstone argued that the G.M.C.'s interest in the idea sprang only from a desire for a 'stepping-stone' towards the prohibition of unqualified practice in the whole medical field. Defending the Home Office's attitude on this head, the Home Secretary, Mr. Ritchie, pointed out that in many towns and villages the only midwives available to the poor were untrained women; if these were forbidden to practise many mothers would receive no assistance at all. Opposing the move for a Select Committee, he urged the House not to ask for too much, but to take 'this modest measure' as it stood. This the House decided to do, granting the second reading without a division.

The Bill was due to be discussed by the Standing Committee on Law in the second week in March. During this stage, by circularizing and lobbying M.P.s, the B.M.A. and the Medical Practitioners' Association strove to get the Bill amended more to their liking. But despite the efforts of M.P.s well disposed to their cause (who, as in 1900, included Lloyd George), the Bill emerged with no material alteration. Attempts to remove the Midwives' Institute's representative from the Central Board, and to substitute one from the Royal British Nurses' Association, failed. A similar fate met efforts to put the Board under the G.M.C., to cut out the Obstetrical Society's certificate as a statutory qualification for registration, to prohibit unqualified practice, and to make the midwife's failure to send for medical aid in difficult cases a criminal offence. Not only this, but participation in the debate by members of the Government had again shown the extent of its support for the Bill. The proposal that the Central Midwives Board should be put under the G.M.C. was firmly resisted by Jesse Collings for the Home Office, and John Burns for the Local Government Board. Stressing that midwives' registration was not merely 'a medical matter', but one which concerned the public interest and involved public finance, they insisted that the formation and oversight of the Board belonged properly to the Government.[13]

As important as the oversight of the Board was its constitution.

Here the interest of the R.B.N.A. was a new development, since only a month before that body had declared that the Bill was one with which it did not wish to be identified.[14] As the Midwives' Institute commented, the R.B.N.A.'s demand was hard to understand, and had certainly not come from the Association's nurse members. In the Institute's view, if there was to be representation for any nursing organization, this should go to the Queen Victoria Jubilee Nursing Institute, which had on its books a considerable number of mid-wives practising in rural areas.[15] The R.B.N.A.'s Charter gave it no duties concerning midwives, and many of its members who were so qualified worked as monthly nurses only. Moreover, Dr. Fardon, the R.B.N.A.'s Secretary—a medical man—had recently acceded to a request of the Medical Defence Union that members holding a midwife's qualification should in future no longer be entered in the R.B.N.A. list as 'midwives', but as 'midwifery nurses'—and all this without their knowledge or consent.

But Mr. O'Connor's eulogy of the R.B.N.A. during the debate on the Bill had let the cat out of the bag. In describing the R.B.N.A. as 'under the control' of medical men he was speaking no more than the truth. The Association was now largely run by the medical members, and its discussion on the Midwives Bill had been carried on almost wholly by them. Furthermore, there were on the R.B.N.A. Council a number of members hostile to the registration of midwives, and to the Obstetrical Society's work in examining them.[16] Any R.B.N.A. representative on the Midwives Board, therefore, might well prove to be an enemy of the midwife and might seek to emphasize the nursing aspect of her work and reduce her role as an independent practitioner.

But the Standing Committee could not be persuaded to equate midwives with nurses. The B.M.A.'s lobbying failed to get the Bill altered, and although Mr. Horsley might complain that it was the action of a leading B.M.A. figure, Dr. Farquharson, in supporting the Bill, which had 'ruined' their efforts, he had to admit that the mood of the House was one of 'extreme irritation' with the medical profession. The *Lancet*, hurt that the profession's 'temperate objections' were regarded as 'narrow and bitter' by the promoters, attributed the Bill's success so far to 'accidental circumstances', and to the lack of a united medical opposition, compared with the 'continuous working and enthusiasm' of its supporters.[17]

What the Bill's medical opponents had failed to realize, however, was that it enjoyed widespread support among the lay public, whereas organized opposition came only from a section of medical men. At last the point had been reached—as the profession had been repeatedly warned it would be—when the matter would be settled

by Parliament without reference to its wishes. Medical opposition
had meant that the Bill could not pass without a vast amount of
support from the general public. Once this existed on a large scale
among their constituents, M.P.s were naturally disinclined to listen
to protests from what they now regarded as merely a sectional
interest. Nor, contrary to the confident expectation of the anti-
midwife party three years before,[18] was the Government prepared
to accept the claim that on this as on other questions, the interests
of the profession were identical with those of the public.

The *Practitioner* had foreseen this clearly, the only medical journal
to do so. The profession, it scolded, had only itself to blame for the
'severe snub' it had received from Parliament and the 'undignified
and odious figure' it had been made to cut before the public. By
allowing an intransigent faction motivated only by a 'narrow and
selfish' spirit to come forward as its spokesmen on platforms, in
medical journals, and on the G.M.C., it had itself been responsible
for the loss of a much better Bill than that which the Government
was now determined to see go through.[19]

Sharing this opinion was the eminent Manchester obstetrician,
Professor W. J. Sinclair, who as a teacher of midwives had himself
been the target of much abuse from the local branch of the B.M.A.
Sinclair maintained that by giving in to the 'anti-midwife agitators'
in the matter of midwives' certificates, the G.M.C. was itself
responsible for Parliament's rejection of its views, in what amounted
to the most 'humiliating' episode in recent medical history. But in
taking the Midwives Board from under the control of the G.M.C.,
the philanthropists and the champions of the emancipation of
women had gone too far. More than any of its predecessors, the Bill
bore the imprint of 'this influential class of women'; in consequence,
it was the 'worst and weakest' yet, and unless amended to give the
G.M.C. general control over the Board, would be 'disastrous' for
the poor whom it aimed to protect.[20]

Yet in spite of all the warnings which the opponents of the Bill
had received about the dangers of asking for too much, the B.M.A.
continued to seek support, not merely for a return to the 1900 Bill,
but for its own more restrictive proposals. Early in June a deputation
of the Association's Council saw the Home Secretary. But Mr.
Ritchie took the line that it was not for the Government to interfere
with a Private Member's measure, the details of which had already
been settled in Committee. He also remained adamant in his
opposition to the prohibition of unqualified practice, and the
deputation perforce concluded that he was in favour of the Bill.[21]

In the meantime, the Obstetrical Society, which of recent years
had not taken an active part in the registration struggle, nevertheless

decided to resist opposition attempts to cut out its certificate as a qualification for registration. In doing so, it wished to defend the interests of the 6,300 women who held this certificate, and also of the Boards of Guardians, hospitals and nursing organizations at home and abroad who over the years had come to demand it as a qualification for midwives in their employ. In a specially prepared pamphlet describing its thirty years' work for the improvement of midwives, the Society pointed out that the majority of its candidates were well-educated and well-trained women, and that it was careful to reject all those who did not come up to the required standard. It would therefore be grossly unfair to impose on these educated women, who had invested time and money in training, the stringent conditions for enrolment envisaged for those who had not.[22]

The Bill reached its report stage in the Commons on 6 June, and there was every indication that the opposition, under the leadership of T. P. O'Connor, would fight it every inch of the way. Sixty-five amendments were down on the order paper, and since there were only three hours at the promoters' disposal, there was a very real danger that the Bill would be talked out. Then, in the course of discussion on an amendment to prohibit the practice 'habitually and for gain' of the unqualified woman, there came a totally unforeseen development. In answer to the Home Secretary's objections that he could not support a measure by which the poor in some country districts would suddenly be deprived of all midwife attendance, Mr. O'Connor suggested that a period of grace might be allowed before the clause was brought into operation. This proposal offered a possible compromise, to which the Home Secretary, although with reluctance, agreed. It was accordingly accepted by Mr. Johnstone for the promoters, and 1910 named as the year in which the prohibition should begin to operate.

Thus, contrary to all expectations, the Commons had shown that they were willing to follow the precedent of the Apothecaries' Act of 1815 and the Pharmacy Act of 1868, rather than that of the Medical and Dentists Acts favoured by the Home Office. More important was the fact that, as a result of Mr. Johnstone's concession, Mr. O'Connor withdrew his opposition to the Bill. Instantly the scene was changed. Whole pages of amendments, mainly in the names of Mr. O'Connor's Irish supporters, were not answered to, and in this atmosphere of relative harmony his proposal that the R.B.N.A. should be represented on the Board was agreed without discussion.

In the Commons the battle was over. During the third reading T. P. O'Connor and another Irishman, Dr. Thompson, took the opportunity to instruct their English colleagues. If only England would follow the Irish example, they argued, there would be no need to fear that the 1910 ban on the unqualified woman would result in a dearth of midwives in country areas; the promoters should therefore press for the adoption at home of the 'well-nigh perfect' Irish dispensary system. The Local Government Board, which was also responsible for the Irish system, had eight years in which to deal with the problem. It would be 'discreditable' if a 'rich country like England' were not willing to follow the example of her poorer neighbour.

The B.M.A. was well pleased with its success in gaining a clause banning unqualified practice, and paid tribute to the 'tact and skill' of T. P. O'Connor.[23] But even O'Connor's eloquence had not been able to persuade the Commons to agree to annual licensing, and the B.M.A. still hoped this might be considered in the Lords. But there, a week later, in an unusually large House in which the atmosphere seemed even more inimical to the profession's views than in the Commons, the Bill received an unopposed second reading. Moreover, during the Committee stage there was a determined attempt to remove the clause prohibiting unqualified practice on the grounds that its operation would produce a scarcity of midwives in rural areas, and that it savoured too much of 'grandmotherly interference with the working classes'. However, this attempt failed, and the clause was retained by a substantial majority.

Other amendments were made, but none involving any important change of principle. The Midwives Board was to be increased by a representative from the Queen's Nursing Institute, as the Midwives' Institute had hoped, thus creating the possibility of a non-medical majority on the Board. Furthermore, the clause requiring the Privy Council to consult with the G.M.C. over the rules of the Midwives Board was opposed as derogatory to the dignity of the Privy Council, and amended to require the Council merely to take account of any representations the G.M.C. might make. All in all, the promoters had good reason to be satisfied with the Bill, which in this form passed its third reading, and on 31 July received the Royal Assent.

At last, after twelve years of almost non-stop controversy within the medical profession, a Midwives Act was on the Statute Book, and the 'midwife question' quietly disappeared from the columns of the medical journals which it had occupied for so long. The *British Medical Journal* regretted, in comparatively mild terms, that the Act did not specify that a majority of members of the Midwives Board should be medical practitioners, but that was all. Indeed, it was not a subject to dwell on, since the Act represented a severe and public humiliation for the G.M.C., the B.M.A., and other medical bodies, at the hands of women's organizations, Parliament, and the Government.

The Midwives' Institute, on the other hand, was triumphant. Although the promoters of successive Midwives Bills had enjoyed the selfless and unwearied service of many medical men—from Aveling and Hart to Humphreys, Cullingworth and Champneys—and of laymen like Pease, Balfour and Johnstone, the success of the 1902 Bill could with justice be described as an achievement by women *for* women.[24] Now, at last, the Institute could take the credit for its twenty years' hard work in the cause of gaining professional status for midwives. Often criticized by women's organizations and journals for not being militant enough in pressing midwives' claims, the Institute had had to face the realities of the situation, while its critics had not. In the event, the 1902 Act gave the midwife a much better position than that proposed in the early Bill of 1890, or the later one of 1900, and the Institute might well congratulate itself on the outcome.

Miss Rosalind Paget, the Institute's Treasurer, took justifiable pleasure in doing this. Replying to the charges of inaction levelled at the Institute by Mrs. Fenwick's *Nursing Record* over the past thirteen years, she asked trained midwives to consider what they owed to the Institute's Council. 'What body of workers have you to thank', she demanded,

> that you are not by law called midwifery or obstetric nurses? That your vested rights in your certificates of training have been considered? That you have a representative on the governing body? That you are not bound hand and foot under those who have only too openly shown how they would 'end' you if they only had the power? Who has worked, unflinchingly, through the hard years of indifference, contempt, suspicion, to a modicum of consideration and respect, in order to create for you a respected and worthy status? . . . you owe all this, and much more, to the Council of the Incorporated Midwives' Institute.[25]

Yet the Act which was to create this 'respected and worthy status', and which was to lay the basis of the present law relating to midwives (as formulated in the Midwives Act 1951), was like no other registration Act, before or since, and was to put midwives in a uniquely disadvantaged position among the professions. First, although conferring State registration on midwives, the Act subjected them to the local authority supervision otherwise associated with the local licensing of tradesmen. Second, although midwives, like other professions, were liable to erasure from the register for professional misconduct, this misconduct was in their case more widely, and more minutely, defined. Moreover, midwives also risked erasure if their *private* lives met with the disapproval of their disciplinary body. Lastly, in contrast with other professions, mid-wives were not to regulate themselves—indeed, a rival profession was to have a dominant voice in their government.

Nonetheless, Miss Paget had been right in her assessment of the Act's significance for midwives. If the campaign for registration had failed, it is unlikely that the drive for the midwife's reinstatement could have been indefinitely sustained. Again, if the Act had sub-jected her to repressive control without conferring compensatory status, as many medical men had hoped it might, it would merely have contributed to her further decline. In either case, she would most probably have vanished from the scene within the next fifty years, squeezed out by her medical competitors. Midwifery would then have become the sole prerogative of what is still, despite the hopes of the nineteenth-century medical woman movement, a pre-dominantly male profession. Women would have suffered a double loss—the disappearance of a traditional female occupation, and the denial of female attendance in childbirth. Finally, from the stand-point of society in general, a medical monopoly of midwifery would have had important implications for the cost of obstetric care, whether financed by private persons, charity, or the State.

That this was not the outcome in England, as it has been in North America, where the midwife has virtually disappeared,[26] is the legacy of those who laboured so long and so hard to keep the office of midwife for women, and whose efforts were crowned in the Midwives Act, 1902.

CHAPTER NINE

Conclusions

In 1902 arrangements were finally made for the regulation of English midwives. This took place fifty to a hundred years after similar steps had been taken by most Continental countries, and taken, moreover, on the initiative of Government itself. In England, where Government only reluctantly allowed itself to become involved in such matters, and where attachment to the principle of Free Trade was much stronger, the impetus for regulation had to come from interested groups who were themselves ready to provide the necessary machinery at no cost to the public. Thus the prospects of any Midwives Bill depended on the strength of the pressure groups behind it and the support they could muster in Parliament.

The Midwives Act had become law ninety years after concrete proposals for midwife regulation had been brought before the Commons in the Associated Apothecaries' omnibus Bill of 1813, and nearly forty years after the subject had appeared on the programme of the Female Medical Society. Of all the categories which the 1813 Bill had proposed to regulate, chemists had been first to obtain a registration Act (in 1852), followed by medical men (after Government intervention) in 1858, and veterinary surgeons in 1881. Dentists, not even mentioned as a distinct group in the 1813 Bill, had been registered with comparatively little fuss by a private member's measure in 1878. Although a permissive clause for the local control of midwives had figured in the Government's unsuccessful Medical Bill of the same year, no Government thereafter had been willing to grasp the nettle of midwife regulation. Hence, when the matter came again before Parliament in 1890, it was as the subject of a private member's Bill, with supporters and opponents on both sides of the House.

Why had it taken so long for a Midwives Act to become law? Hopes that the 1878 Dentists Act would serve as a precedent for a private member's Bill on midwives had been sorely disappointed.

Though dentistry and midwifery were similar in their relation to medicine in that both dentists and midwives shared their field with medical practitioners, dentistry, unlike midwifery, did not provide a way into general practice. There had thus been no great medical opposition to the elevation of dentists to professional status, which was in any case to be subject to medical supervision through the G.M.C. The G.M.C. had therefore no reason for declining to undertake their regulation. However, the G.M.C.'s unfortunate experiences with dentists' registration had made it reluctant to embark on what might prove a larger and even more difficult task—and one which, moreover, some of its members considered to be below its dignity. Furthermore, the case of midwives was complicated by the anti-feminism prevalent among medical practitioners, many of whom demanded that women should not only be kept out of medicine, but, as soon as economic conditions allowed, driven from midwifery as well.

Yet another difficulty lay in the nature of the great body of midwives themselves. Agitation for professional registration comes usually from activists within an occupation and is a measure of its growing strength and organization. Midwives, however, numbered within their ranks only a few women of education and status who were vocal enough and influential enough to press for a registration Bill. The overwhelming majority were poor, untrained, irregular workers, who included a large number of women who could neither read nor write—such are not the stuff of which a successful pressure group is made. It was for this reason that the few midwives able to take up the matter depended so heavily on the goodwill and initiative of leading medical men in the same field. It was these men who, along with lay supporters drawn from the aristocracy and upper middle classes, had prestige and power enough to defeat the militant opposition arising from the ranks of the socially inferior general practitioner. In the more egalitarian society of North America, however, where the rank and file of the medical profession was (and still is) more powerful than in this country, the midwife has been driven into virtual extinction.

But their dependence on medical help made the midwives' road to registration a hazardous one. The Midwives' Institute aimed at making midwifery a suitable profession for educated women, and sought State registration as a means to that end. The medical side of the movement, on the other hand, though wishing to see a body of adequately trained women available for work among the poor, were at the same time anxious to restrict their independence and make them clearly subordinate to the medical profession. Thus the price paid for State registration was a substantial degree of medical control, and in acceding to this the London-based Midwives' Institute had met bitter criticism from militant provincial midwives preferring no registration at all to the system proposed. It was for the same reason that Midwives Bills had lacked the general support of the women's rights movements, since many women's leaders viewed the campaign's proposals as yet another attempt by men to limit the work of women in the interests of their male competitors. Finally, its supporters had been opposed by nurses seeking their own Act—a group from which midwives might reasonably have expected most help.

Faced with all this opposition, the only way open to the promoters of this private member's Bill was to gain public support on a scale hitherto unprecedented for the enactment into law of a professional registration measure, and it was largely through the hard work of women themselves that this support had been won. It was middle-class 'ladies' like Mrs. Smith and Miss Paget, who, coming into midwifery from the already respectable calling of nursing, had laboured over the years to make their new field an acceptable one for educated women to enter. Again, it was women who had organized the campaign for public and Parliamentary support which had made victory possible. The Act, as the Midwives' Institute was quick to point out, was a great triumph for women, who, though voteless themselves, had nevertheless carried their views in Parliament. Further, the long years of neglect by that all-male body of this 'woman's question' was yet another compelling argument for the enfranchisement of women.[1]

The Act was also of great significance to the medical profession. Though the President of the G.M.C., Sir William Turner, took comfort in the fact that it protected the rights of the medical profession from encroachment by the midwife,[2] it could not be disguised that both the G.M.C. and the B.M.A. had suffered a signal defeat at the hands of Parliament. Yet the Act had given the medical profession a very large say in midwives' affairs. Local supervision was to be in the hands of Medical Officers of Health, and although membership of the Central Midwives Board was not required to be entirely medical, the Board, by contrast with the more recently established registration bodies for nurses, dentists, and other professions supplementary to medicine, has always had a medical majority.

More remarkable, the Board was not actually required to include even one member of the body of workers whose practice it was to regulate. It was only because of the Privy Council's right to nominate a woman, and the fortuitous representation on the Board of two nursing organizations, that any midwives were in fact appointed.

Though the justice of appointing midwives as such to the Board was finally recognized in 1920, they were at the same time statutorily precluded (as they still are) from becoming a majority of the membership, and it was not until 1973 that a midwife became Chairman of the Board. While other professions are governed by bodies including a majority (at least) of their own members, midwives have the unenviable distinction of being the only profession controlled by a body on which its members must never be more than a minority. Users of midwife services, however, have had even less representation, and the appointment to the Board of a woman who has borne children has been a very rare occurrence.

The matter of midwife representation on the Board was of vital importance to midwives. First, there was the very real danger that medical jealousy might keep the standard of their training unduly low, and its scope unduly limited. This danger was very clearly illustrated when the Board's rules were first drawn up in 1903. Although *Nursing Notes* found these rules 'very stringent for the midwife and very tender to the susceptibilities of the medical man', they were not limiting enough for three of the Board's medical members. Midwives, they argued, should not be taught the treatment for haemorrhages, nor the management or feeding of infants after the first ten days—a view in which they were supported by the *British Medical Journal*. Yet, as both *Nursing Notes* and the *Lancet* pointed out, in many areas the nearest doctor might be miles away, and surely a midwife should know how to deal with emergencies? As for infant feeding, said *Nursing Notes*, a country mother would no more consult the doctor than the parson, especially as it would cost her half-a-crown for the privilege.[3]

Thus the Board's disciplinary powers were more extensive than those granted to the regulatory body of any other profession. It was the Board's duty to lay down a strict and comprehensive code of conduct governing the midwife's practice. The rules made by the Board outlined in minute detail the midwife's duties to mother and child at the birth and during the ensuing ten days, even laying down requirements as to the dress she was to wear, the appliances she was to carry, the records she was to keep, the number of times she was to visit the mother, and in what circumstances she was to send for a doctor. Since infringements of these rules rendered the midwife liable to erasure from the Roll, she was far more vulnerable than were doctors or dentists to action from the G.M.C. The G.M.C. had no power to concern itself with such details and in any case left complaints of negligence and malpractice on the part of doctors and dentists to be brought before the Courts.

Another unique feature of the Act was its requirement that the expenses of the Central Midwives Board should in part be met by the ratepayer—a recognition of the inability of midwives to finance unaided the machinery of their professional registration.[4] This made midwives the only profession whose registration was subsidized by the ratepayers, an arrangement which continued until the re-organization of the National Health Service in 1974 laid the health duties of County Councils on the new Area Health Authorities.

In other respects, however, the Act served as an important precedent. Not only did it set the stage for the Nurses Act of 1919, but, as its general practitioner opponents had feared, for the eventual State registration, among other occupations, of the optician, the masseuse, and the lowly corn-cutter. With opticians, who in 1906 were the next group to seek registration, the medical opposition was more successful than it had been with midwives. Using the same arguments as had been used against midwife registration, and earlier, against that of chemists, they were able to delay the registra-tion of opticians—an 'inferior and purely commercial order of medical practitioners', as the G.M.C. described them—for over fifty years. Not until 1958 did opticians finally gain their Act, followed shortly afterwards by the other two categories, now calling themselves 'physiotherapists', and 'chiropodists'—all as a result of Government action. However, the attempts of those other com-petitors of the medical profession, the bone-setters, or 'osteopaths', to gain registration have so far failed.

In prohibiting practice by the uncertified midwife the Act had followed the Apothecaries Act of 1815 and the Pharmacy Act of 1868, rather than the Acts registering doctors, dentists or veterinary surgeons. The pressure for this ban had not come from midwives themselves but from members of a rival profession, and although justified by its advocates as being in the public interest, it was con-fidently expected to pay handsome dividends to the medical pro-fession itself. One advantage looked for in militant medical quarters was the precedent the Act would provide for the amendment of the Medical Acts to prohibit unqualified medical practice, a prohibition obtaining in France and elsewhere on the Continent. But although this medical hope was never realized, the Act did serve as a precedent in this respect for the revised schemes for dentists and for veterinary surgeons,[5] and for the registration of opticians when this was finally achieved in 1958.

To the medical man fearing the midwife's competition a more immediate advantage of the ban on the uncertified woman lay in the fact that in future all new midwives must take the Board's examina-tion. Hence, unless the Midwives Board was willing to risk denuding large areas of the country of midwives, the standard of qualification could not be allowed to rise beyond the capabilities of the average recruit. Registration was thus unlikely to produce in significant numbers the highly skilled midwife who might well prove a competitor for the best-paid midwifery practice. Despite the medical opposition's complaints that the Act would create an 'inferior order' of medical practitioners, the ban on unqualified practice was the best guarantee that the spectre which had haunted the medical profession for so long could not materialize in the person of the certified midwife.

As expected, the Board initially required candidates for its examination to have had only three months' approved training. Although the Board had no responsibility for the supply of midwives, it would not have been realistic at the outset for it to have specified a longer period. Later on, and in stages, training was lengthened to two years[6] as the standard of candidates improved. Eventually, the time arrived—as the Act's promoters, and, indeed, their opponent Mrs. Fenwick, had hoped—when the majority of practising midwives were also trained nurses.

The Act's promoters had often been twitted by Mrs. Fenwick for their lack of vision in accepting a requirement of only three months' training for the new registered midwife, yet their appreciation of the economic realities of the situation proved more accurate than hers. In accordance with her ideals, the length of training laid down for registered nurses under the 1919 Act was set at three years, the level of the most highly trained in the occupation. However, as other opportunities for the middle-class girl who she hoped would ultimately constitute the bulk of the profession continued to expand, this became an increasingly unrealistic ideal. Twenty years later, in 1943, a subordinate class of nurses with a shorter training was created, in order that a sufficient supply of trained workers could be maintained in the field.

What was the body of workers which the newly established Midwives Board was called on to regulate? The Midwives Roll of 1905 contained no less than 22,308 names, of whom 7,465 held the Obstetrical Society's certificate, 2,322 held hospital certificates, and 12,521 were midwives in 'bona fide' practice who held no certificate at all. Many of these were totally illiterate and had to have the records and forms demanded under the Board's rules filled in for them. Some also had difficulty in reading a clinical thermometer, and one old midwife regularly took hers to the parson to have it read. Not all who enrolled actually practised, some being nurses who merely wished to register their midwifery qualification. Those who did practise attended probably about half of all births in the country. A small proportion worked for hospitals and maternity charities or rural nursing associations; the great majority, however, practised on their own account, delivering their patients at home, where all but a tiny fraction of births took place.

However, in the event not all practising midwives were required to observe the Board's rules in their entirety. Soon after commencing operations the Board had incurred the hostility of Poor Law Infirmaries for its 'autocratic' rulings on the conditions it required should be satisfied by those institutions to be approved as midwife training schools.[7] Despite the Board's objections, the Privy Council acceded to the request of the Local Government Board that these institutions be exempted from the Board's rules, an exemption which remained in force until 1924.

As was to be expected, the duty of seeing that midwives kept the Board's minutely detailed rules was discharged by different local authorities with varying degrees of interest and efficiency. Some big authorities, like London and Manchester, appointed well-qualified inspectors who did good work in gaining the co-operation of the untrained 'bona fide' midwives by instructing them in the Board's rules, showing them how to take antiseptic precautions, and how to read a thermometer. In many areas, however, the work of inspection was left to persons without suitable qualifications. These were commonly health visitors, women generally of higher social status than midwives, but with little or no practical experience of midwifery, who in consequence were resented by midwives as ignorant and overbearing. In some areas the duty was laid on the sanitary inspector, who came to it 'straight from rubbish tips and drains', in others, on the poorly remunerated Medical Officer of Health himself, 'who had forgotten most of the midwifery he had ever learnt', or even on his clerk. Occasionally it was given to the over-burdened superintendent of the local nursing association. In many rural areas, however, the strict enforcement of the rules was un-realistic, and as the opponents of the prohibitory clause had forecast would have cleared these districts of midwives altogether. There, in default of a policy for the provision of trained midwives on a sub-sidized or salaried basis, only the 'gentlest' administration of the Act was possible.

On the other hand, some local authorities used their powers to harass midwives rather than to encourage their improvement. It might have been that the Medical Officer of Health was himself hostile to midwives, or that the supervising committee included a number of similarly minded medical men, all in practice in the area. The power of the supervising authority to suspend from practice a midwife who had had a case of puerperal fever in order to prevent the spread of infection presented a ready opportunity for such harassment. Cases were known where midwives were suspended for far longer than was necessary for purposes of disinfection—sometimes for weeks—or even months—in contravention of the spirit of the Act and, of course, without compensation for practice lost as a result.[8] The vindictiveness with which certain local authorities used these supervisory powers justified the insistence of the Act's promoters on leaving the final say in disciplinary matters to the Central Board.

In the early years of the Act's operation the number of midwives brought before the Board increased steadily as local supervisory authorities stepped up their implementation of the Act. In addition to more serious breaches of the rules women were struck off for failure to wear a washing dress, carry the required appliances and keep proper records. However, as the number of 'bona fide' midwives gradually declined, so did the penal cases brought before the Board. By the 1930s, it was apparent that to subject the now better educated and trained midwife to the precise detailed code of rules designed for the control of the untrained woman of the past was incompatible with the now accepted national policy of raising the status of the occupation and in 1947 the rules were revised to take account of the changed situation.

Initially the Board was equally stringent in its attitude to the midwife's general conduct, and a number of women were struck off whose only offence was that they had 'lapsed from the path of virtue'. In taking this line the Board had the warm approval of *Nursing Notes*, the journal of the Midwives' Institute. Reporting the High Court case of Stocks v. the Central Midwives Board, the journal had been 'aggrieved' that Mrs. Stocks had won her appeal against the Board's decision to strike her off for 'immorality'.[9] The facts were that Mrs. Stocks' husband had left her some years earlier with two children to keep, that she had subsequently formed a union with another man, and had a child by him. However, she had only won her appeal on a procedural irregularity in the Board's handling of her case, and the Court had upheld the Board's right to strike a midwife off on these grounds—a power which it still retains under the Act currently governing midwife practice, the Midwives Act of 1951. Though nowadays the Board does not generally concern itself with a midwife's private life, it may still erase a woman's name from the Roll for some conduct not directly connected with her work if it considers that to allow such conduct would bring the profession into disrepute. Thus the Board still exercises stricter control over midwives than that wielded by their respective governing bodies over all other professions, with the exception of nurses—significantly, a predominantly female occupation.[10]

But the Board could only discipline the certified midwife; the prevention of unqualified practice lay in the hands of local authorities and the Courts. In this respect the Act contained a curious anomaly. Although practice by the uncertified woman was forbidden, that of the unqualified man was not, and it was not until 1926 that this loop-hole was closed. The uncertified 'handy woman', however, still practised widely, preferred because of her relative cheapness, her willingness to help around the house and, in some cases, because of her 'churchyard luck'. Many local authorities were dilatory in prosecuting such women, and even when they did, their efforts were often thwarted by the difficulty of proving 'habitual' practice and by the refusal of magistrates to take the law seriously. Moreover, in some country areas there was a shortage of certified midwives, and to have prevented the 'handywoman' from practising would have left local mothers with no assistance whatsoever.

In many cases, too, general practitioners aided and abetted the uncertified woman by 'covering' her attendance. In return for part of the fee, the practitioner would represent the case as his own for the purpose of any legal formalities, which in later years included the notification of the birth and the signing of the maternity benefit form under the 1911 Insurance Act. Such conduct enabled the uncertified woman (who was no threat to the doctor's better paying practice) to flourish at the expense of the certified midwife, whose competition he feared. Although in 1916 the G.M.C. at last began to take action against this type of 'covering', it still continued, and it was for this reason that the Act of 1936 barred the uncertified woman from acting even as a maternity nurse.[11]

The hostility of some general practitioners towards the certified midwife had shown itself in a variety of ways. When the Roll was first set up some had tried to frighten midwives out of registering. Again, there was still the old problem of who should pay the doctor called in by the midwife in an emergency. Under the rules of the Central Midwives Board the midwife was required to call in a doctor to difficult and dangerous cases, but there was no provision for his payment—any more than there was for hers. Not surprisingly, this did nothing to improve relations, and often the midwife was forced to pay the fee out of her own pocket if she wished a doctor to attend. In some areas doctors banded together, as in 1901 the Swanscombe doctors had done, refusing to attend midwives' emergency calls, on the plea that any consequent fatalities would be justified if they contributed to the early disappearance of midwives. Indeed, as evidence to the 1909 Departmental Enquiry into the Act's working showed, in some districts pressure from general practitioners was strong enough to prevent local nursing associations from employing midwives acting on their own responsibility, thus forcing patients to engage a doctor in every case.

In 1913 this question was again brought to the public notice by the death of a woman in Cheshunt in Hertfordshire. Three Cheshunt doctors, all members of the Enfield Medico-Ethical Society, had refused to attend a midwife's emergency call in consequence of a prior agreement that no member of the Society would attend such cases without immediate payment of a higher fee than usual—a guinea and a half. In this case the midwife had sent to each of the doctors in turn a letter informing them that the mother was insured with the Hearts of Oak Friendly Society, and that the fee would ultimately be forthcoming, but all refused to attend. The patient died, and the doctors in question were censured by the jury at the subsequent inquest.[12]

Ever since the 1902 Act had come into operation, the proportion of cases in which midwives sent for the doctor had been rising steadily, but it was not until the Midwives Act of 1918 that the vexed question of who should pay his fee was at last decided. Under the Act local supervising authorities were required to pay the fee whenever the patient's family was unable to do so, and were empowered to recover it where possible later. From this time on, relations between midwives and general practitioners, though often still leaving a great deal to be desired, began to improve.

This improvement continued, despite an increase in the proportion of births attended by midwives from the 50% officially estimated in 1909 to an average of 60% or so throughout the country in the 1930s.[13] However, the consequent decrease in the general practitioner's share in midwifery was less the result of midwife registration than of two other unrelated factors. One was the 1914–18 war, which had drained off many doctors to the front, and the other was the 1911 National Insurance Act, which, by providing general practitioner services to insured workers earning under £160 p.a., for the first time had given the poorer medical man some degree of financial security. General practitioners were thus less anxious to continue with 'cheap' midwifery, which, though still time-consuming, gave a comparatively poor return, and which, for attendance on National Insurance patients, required compliance with the exacting conditions of the scheme's regulations. Indeed, such was the improvement in the general practitioner's position that the 1936 Act establishing a salaried local authority midwife service—the bogey with which Dr. Rentoul had sought to frighten the profession forty years before—passed without adverse comment in the medical press.

As the old antagonisms began to wane, other changes took place which were of equal importance to the midwife. Fears for the nation's security had led to growing concern with the breeding of a healthy race, capable of defending homeland and Empire. This preoccupation had weakened older objections to State provision of maternity services other than through the deterrent and stigmatizing Poor Law. In the years just before the 1914–18 war there had been a great change of outlook at the Local Government Board, which had begun to grant-aid local authority schemes for salaried or subsidized midwife services, a development further encouraged by the new Ministry of Health from its establishment in 1919. It was this new attitude which facilitated the partial solution to the problem of who should pay the doctor called in to midwives' cases through payment by the local authority. Even here, however, old fears of encouraging the poor to depend on the rates led many local authorities to adopt a strict attitude towards recovery of the fee, which often meant subjecting the patient's family to humiliating enquiries at a time when she might not yet have recovered from a difficult birth.[14]

By now the 1902 Act was beginning to bear fruit. With each year that passed trained midwives constituted a larger proportion of those in practice, and the number of 'bona-fide' midwives allowed onto the Roll in 1905 rapidly declined. Yet even as late as the 1930s the practice of the illegal uncertificated woman still continued in many areas. In some country districts there was no certificated midwife; in others the 'handywoman' was often preferred because of her cheapness and her willingness to help about the house.[15]

However, the standards of practice by the trained midwife were not always all that they should have been. Such shortcomings were less likely to occur in the practice of the salaried midwife responsible to her employing body, than in that of the independent woman working on her own account.[16] It was also more difficult to enlist the co-operation of the independent midwife in the arrangements for ante- and post-natal care increasingly fostered by local authorities in their efforts to provide a complete maternity service. Indeed, such co-operation worked against the midwife's own interests. A poor patient was unlikely to pay more for such care and any referral to a doctor or ante-natal clinic for further examination might result in the loss of the patient—and her fee—to the doctor himself, or to the hospital.

There were other developments, too, which were unfavourable to the independent midwife. Though the coming of National Insurance had made it easier for her to obtain a higher fee, and had reduced the number of bad debts, her general position was steadily becoming less and less tenable. A number of factors had played a part in this decline. One was the continuing fall in the birth-rate, which at 15 per 1,000 of the population was now only half what it had been in the 1890s. Another had been the success of Government policy in encouraging local authorities to establish, either directly or through grant-aiding voluntary organizations, a subsidized or wholly salaried midwife service. At the same time the increasing emphasis on the need for improved midwifery education for both midwives and doctors had led hospitals concerned in their training to seek more and more cases, both as out- and in-patients, for their instruction. With the transfer in 1930 of the Poor Law Infirmaries to the County Councils and the consequent removal of the stigma associated with these institutions, the proportion of hospital births had begun to grow rapidly, increasing from 15% in 1927 to over 34% ten years later.[17] Even without this latest development, the 1929 Departmental Committee studying the employment of midwives found that although a few with extensive practices might earn more than £275 p.a., a very large number practising full-time earned only £90–£120.[18]

In deciding to establish a whole-time salaried midwife service the Government was primarily concerned with the seemingly intractable problem of maternal mortality. Despite the high hopes nursed by advocates of the 1902 Act, the maternal mortality rate had remained almost stationary. During the thirty odd years since the passing of the Act the general death rate had fallen by one third, and the infant mortality rate had been halved. Yet, as Table I shows, although there had been an appreciable fall in the maternal mortality rate in the years immediately following the 1902 Act, this had not been sustained. Worse still, from 1928 it had shown a significant rise, climbing again to an average of over 4 per 1,000 live births. Even more puzzling, maternal mortality was lower among the poor than among the better-off.[19]

Maternal mortality is influenced by many factors, including the age and physique of the mother and the number of children she has already borne, besides the skill of her attendant. However, the series of Ministry of Health investigations conducted during the inter-war years demonstrated clearly that lack of skill or knowledge in the attendant doctor or midwife, both before and after delivery, was the single most important factor.[20] Yet there was no doubt that the gradual replacement of the old 'bona fide' midwife by the trained woman had resulted in a great improvement in the general standard of midwife practice. As the Act's promoters had predicted, the trained midwife was more ready to send for medical aid in difficult births, and the proportion of cases in which the doctor was called in had steadily increased. There had been a steady increase, too, in the proportion of midwives working on a salaried or subsidized basis for

Table I

England and Wales. Mortality of Women from Puerperal Causes in Childbirth per 1,000 children born alive, 1891–1934

(From Table LXXXII of the Registrar-General's Statistical Review for 1934, Text volume, page 124.)

Classification in use before 1911

Quinquennial Rates, 1891–1930				Annual Rates, 1911–1934			
Years	Puerperal Sepsis	Other Puerperal Causes	Total Puerperal Mortality	Year	Puerperal Sepsis	Other Puerperal Causes	Total Puerperal Mortality
1891–95	2·60	2·89	5·49	1911	1·52	2·15	3·67
				1912	1·47	2·31	3·78
1896–1900	2·12	2·57	4·69	1913	1·34	2·37	3·71
				1914	1·63	2·32	3·95
1901–05	1·95	2·32	4·27	1915	1·56	2·38	3·94
1906–10	1·56	2·18	3·74	1916	1·47	2·40	3·87
				1917	1·39	2·27	3·66
1911–15	1·50	2·31	3·81	1918	1·35	2·20	3·55
				1919	1·76	2·36	4·12
1916–20	1·59	2·29	3·88	1920	1·87	2·25	4·12
1921–25	1·48	2·21	3·69	1921	1·46	2·25	3·71
				1922	1·46	2·12	3·58
1926–30	1·78	2·23	4·01	1923	1·38	2·22	3·60
				1924	1·48	2·22	3·70
				1925	1·62	2·24	3·86
				1926	1·64	2·23	3·87
				1927	1·63	2·20	3·83
				1928	1·85	2·30	4·15
				1929	1·83	2·24	4·07
				1930	1·96	2·19	4·16
				1931	1·71	2·22	3·93
				1932	1·68	2·33	4·01
				1933	1·90	2·42	4·32
				1934	2·10	2·30	4·39

Table II

Mortality, per 1,000 Live Births, of Married Women according to Social Class of Husband—England and Wales, 1930-32

(Table 18, Ministry of Health, *Report on an Investigation into Maternal Mortality*, 1937, p. 302.)

Cause No.	Cause	Classes I & II	Class III	Class IV	Class V	All married women
140–150	All puerperal causes	4·44	4·11	4·16	3·89	4·13
142–150	Puerperal causes other than abortion	3·94	3·55	3·60	3·32	3·58
142, 143	Ectopic gestation and other accidents of pregnancy ...	0·17	0·15	0·16	0·12	0·15
144	Puerperal haemorrhage ...	0·50	0·44	0·48	0·60	0·49
145	Puerperal sepsis	1·45	1·33	1·21	1·16	1·29
146, 147	Albuminuria and other toxaemias	0·81	0·81	0·85	0·68	0·79
148	Phlegmasia alba dolens ...	0·40	0·30	0·32	0·26	0·31
149	Other accidents of childbirth	0·52	0·42	0·46	0·40	0·44

maternity charities, nursing associations, hospital out-patient departments, or—a more recent development—local authorities. By 1936 these women constituted half of the 16,000 practising midwives on the Roll. Many of their patients were over-burdened, undernourished, and living in insanitary conditions, and, in country areas, far from specialist aid, yet many of the organizations employing salaried midwives, as Sir Kingsley Wood, the Conservative Minister of Health, pointed out when introducing the 1936 Midwives Bill, averaged a maternal death-rate of only half, or less than half, the national rate.[21] It was not these midwives who were responsible for the continuing high death-rate among childbearing women.

It may be, of course, that too much had been expected of the 1902 Act, and that the old untrained midwife had never been responsible for as much mortality as had been attributed to her—an opinion strongly maintained at the time by feminist critics of successive Midwives Bills. That there had always been a large number of women who were grossly incompetent was never in doubt. But, as defenders of the midwife had pointed out for over two hundred

years, many medical men practising obstetrics were equally inadequate for the work, and for much the same reasons. Midwifery
training for many medical students was still very deficient, and the
calls of general practice were, as always, diverse and pressing. In
these circumstances it was not surprising that the old charge of
'meddlesome midwifery' was now echoed with monotonous regular-
ity in the series of Ministry of Health reports on maternal mortality
which appeared in the inter-war years.

Too often, the Ministry's investigations recorded, there was unnecessary and premature application of the forceps, and many
doctors neglected to take antiseptic precautions. Again, some preferred the unqualified handywoman—herself often innocent of the
need for antiseptic measures—to assist them in their cases rather
than the qualified midwife or maternity nurse. Despite the increased
emphasis on the need for ante-natal care, some practitioners did not
provide this service and others again objected if their patients
received it from the local authority clinic or elsewhere.[22]

Ironically, the very fact that trained midwives sent for medical
assistance in a greater proportion of cases may in itself provide the
clue to the maternal mortality puzzle. As Fairbairn found from his
analysis of the records of the Queen's Institute's midwives for the
twenty years between 1905 and 1925, the rise in the proportion of
cases to which midwives called the doctor was not accompanied by
the expected decrease in the maternal death-rate. On the contrary,
the death-rate actually rose in step with it.[23] It may be therefore that
any benefit resulting from the improvement in midwifery practice
was offset by a decline in standards of midwifery in general practice.
For years now general practitioners had been steadily relinquishing
their ordinary cases to midwives. This factor, together with the
falling birth-rate and the growing trend towards institutional
delivery meant that in many areas general practitioners lacked that
experience of attending normal labours which is a necessary preliminary to the proper understanding and treatment of abnormal
ones.[24] Just as in Margaret Stephen's day, the doctor called in to an
emergency might have been chosen less for his obstetric skill than for
his proximity or his cheapness.

The greatest number of errors leading to a fatal termination were,
as the 1930 Departmental Committee on Maternal Mortality and
Morbidity pointed out, inevitably attributable to doctors, since in
difficult cases the midwife was required by the Board's rules to send
for a doctor, and the responsibility for the outcome rested with him.[25]
However, the Committee concluded that deaths following abnormal
labour would only fall when general practitioners had realized that
the conditions of the ordinary working-class home were not suitable

for the performance of obstetric operations which would tax the skill of experienced obstetricians in well-equipped hospitals. Since it would never be possible to make an expert obstetrician of every medical student, any more than to make him a surgeon, it followed that abnormal cases should be sent to hospital. For attendance in normal cases the Committee recommended the extension of the employment of midwives as an essential condition of a satisfactory service.[26]

The Midwives Act 1936 was, as Parliament realized, a 'pre-war measure'. National concern over the falling birth-rate and the apprehension of future war were strong enough to overcome old individualist objections to 'State midwifery' and to allow a Conservative Government to propose the Bill, and the House to pass it, as an agreed measure. Under the Act local authorities were to ensure a salaried whole-time midwife service, adequate to local needs, which would provide the services of a certificated midwife free or at reduced cost, and thus solve the old problem of furnishing qualified attendance to the poor, and especially to inhabitants of remote country areas. The Act also provided for the local authority midwife to be engaged as a maternity nurse in cases where the general practitioner was in charge of the delivery. The object of this provision was to render unnecessary the employment of the unqualified handywoman, who was banned from attending childbirth in any capacity.

Like the 1902 Act, the Act of 1936 was a landmark in the professional development of midwives. Those working in the new service would be granted a better living, with better conditions and prospects than were generally available to the independent midwife, who had hitherto suffered all the discipline of local authority service without any of its rewards. These new arrangements would, it was hoped, raise the status of midwifery and attract more educated women to the profession. But in recognition of the loss which remaining independent midwives would further sustain from the competition of the cheaper local authority services, the Act provided for the compensation of all those willing to withdraw from practice within a given period, even allowing local authorities to retire compulsorily those whom they considered incapacitated for the work.[27]

By creating a salaried service in which the midwife was the employee of the local health authority, the Act greatly facilitated the extension of her work into the vital field of ante-natal care. It also accelerated the provision of analgesia in domiciliary midwifery,[28] so far only available to the patients of the medical practitioner. Finally, since local authorities now had to take responsibility for providing an adequate supply of certificated midwives for their area, it was at last realistic for the Central Midwives Board to extend the training to be required of future entrants to the profession to two years for those without nurse training, and to require periodic attendances at refresher courses from those already in practice. From now on the great majority of midwives would be salaried professionals, offering a more complete service and at last receiving public recognition of the value of their work to the national well-being.

But the new midwife owed much of her improved status to thirty years' hard work by the Central Midwives Board, a fortuitously constituted body representing conflicting interests and established in the face of strong medical opposition, which in 1902 had embarked on an entirely new venture in professional registration. However, such was the wise guidance of its first Chairman, Dr. Francis Champneys, that in a few years the Board had gone a long way towards raising the standing of the hitherto despised midwife, at the same time greatly adding to the goodwill with which the Act was regarded by responsible medical opinion.[29]

Yet the Board had not always had the support it might have expected from the government departments—first the Local Government Board and later the Ministry of Health—charged with supervision of health matters. In 1919 the oversight of the Board, together with that of the new Nursing Council, was transferred from the Privy Council to the newly created Ministry of Health. From the first the Ministry was determined to exercise tighter control over the Board than that wielded by the Privy Council. Accordingly, when, a few years later, the Board asked permission to inspect midwife training arrangements in Poor Law Infirmaries its request was dismissed as 'impertinent'[30] by Ministry officials and as soon as the opportunity arose, the Ministry appointed one of its permanent officials to the Board. Relations between the two bodies were never harmonious, but the crucial trial of strength came in 1929 with the report of the Ministry's Departmental Committee on the Training and Employment of Midwives. Although only one organization had given evidence in favour of such a step, a majority of the Committee, whose membership was heavily weighted towards health administration, reported in favour of severely curtailing the Board's functions.[31] Responsibility for training, including determination of the curriculum and inspection of training schools, was to be transferred to the Ministry itself. Not only would the Ministry continue to inspect its Poor Law training schools, but its inspectors, whose qualifications the Board had previously called into question, would now also inspect training schools at the most prestigious lying-in hospitals. Thus the tables were turned on the Board's consultant obstetricians who had been so critical of Ministry policies in the past. Examinations and disciplinary matters were to be handed over to a rump Board, on which the B.M.A. and the Society of Medical Officers of Health were to be represented, but the Royal Colleges, representing obstetricians, and the Midwives' Institute, representing midwives, were not.

In this way the professional development of midwives would have been placed largely in the hands of the Ministry and local health authorities. These, as supervisors and employers of midwives, would have been in an increasingly powerful position, especially if the Committee's main proposal for a national maternity service had gone through. Consultant obstetricians, who had played such an important part in midwife training over the years, were to be excluded, as indeed, were midwives themselves. These recommendations were, of course, highly satisfactory to the Ministry, which looked forward to no longer being 'hampered' by the Board's inconvenient views.[32] As was to be expected, the Committee's scheme was opposed by the Board, which, arguing from past experience of Ministry laxity over training in Poor Law infirmaries, held that a general decline in training standards would inevitably follow. Opposition also came from midwives who were seeking to gain the same control over their regulation as was enjoyed by other professions, and from medical men who feared the encroachment of the Ministry in their own professional affairs. In the event, however, the current economic crisis prevented the adoption of the Committee's recommendation for a comprehensive state maternity scheme, and the accompanying proposals for the Board's reconstruction were quietly allowed to die. Since then there has been no further threat to the Board's position, which was confirmed in the Midwives Act of 1951.[33] However, as the Board itself observed in its 1971 Report, there are still problems inherent in a situation in which the Government department charged with the oversight of a profession is an interested party in its affairs.

But whatever the Board had achieved, the midwife's new status would not have been won without the watchful determination exercised on her behalf by the Midwives' Institute, which over the previous thirty years had laboured long and hard to complete the work which the 1902 Act had begun. At last, in 1935, the value to the nation of the Institute's work was officially recognized by the award of the order of Dame of the British Empire to Miss Rosalind Paget, who had devoted so much of her long life to the midwives' cause. In 1941, sixty years after its humble beginnings as the tiny Matrons' Aid Society, the Midwives' Institute itself was honoured with its own Charter. The 'Colledg of Midwifes' dreamed of by

Elizabeth Cellier two and a half centuries before had finally become a reality. One further privilege remained to be conferred. In 1947, the year in which the last 'bona fide' midwife enrolled under the 1902 Act ceased to practise, the College was granted the prefix 'Royal'. The 'fine profession' to which Miss Jane Wilson had looked forward in 1902 had at last come of age.

But this is not the end of the story. At the same time other changes were taking place which were to have equal, or even greater significance for the midwife's future role. In establishing a framework for the development of midwifery as a profession, the sponsors of the 1902 Act had hoped that in the new certificated midwife poor women would find a safe attendant for ordinary childbirth at a price they could afford. Yet in failing to make provision for the supply of trained midwives, or, indeed, for medical attendance in abnormal cases, the Act had merely offered a nineteenth-century individualist response to a problem only susceptible of a twentieth-century collectivist solution. The local authority midwifery service set up under the 1936 Act was, however, only a stage on the way towards this solution. In 1939 came the Second World War—like the first, a powerful catalyst of social change. After the war, the new determination to attack social problems on a national scale led, among other things, to the establishment of the National Health Service which offered free and comprehensive health care to the whole population. For the first time the services of the midwife, the general practitioner, and the hospital were free to all women, whatever their income or social class, and for the first time the choice of attendant and the scope of maternity care for each patient could be made on medical rather than financial grounds.

As might have been expected, the new arrangements, which removed the economic barrier between patient and doctor and guaranteed the payment of practitioners undertaking obstetric care, whether or not they actually attended the delivery, led to a rise in the proportion of midwifery cases in which general practitioners were engaged. Initially this led to resentment, sometimes amounting to open hostility, among midwives who had been accustomed to sole responsibility for their patients, and who, in cases where medical aid was required, had sent for the practitioner of their own choice. Though this resentment gradually diminished as doctors and midwives became more accustomed to working together as colleagues rather than competitors, the continuing and officially encouraged trend to hospital delivery (in some areas now almost 100%) has meant that this resurgence of interest in midwifery on the part of the general practitioner could not be sustained. The number of general practitioner maternity units is declining, and the position may soon be reached when the separation of midwifery from general practice advocated by Dr. James Edmunds a hundred years ago, will, as far as the actual delivery is concerned, be complete.

This trend to hospital delivery has brought great changes to the midwifery profession. Although at the great majority of deliveries the midwife is still the senior person present, in the move from home to hospital she has lost some of her status as an independent practitioner. At the same time she has also lost the continuing contact with the mother and family which in home midwifery lasted at least ten days and gave her a large part of the satisfaction to be gained from her work. Domiciliary midwives who receive their patients from hospital after early discharge may have time to establish this relationship, but have been robbed of the midwife's chief function— of attending the delivery—and may feel themselves in consequence little more than maternity nurses, as are their North American counterparts.

It is in keeping with these developments that the report of the Committee set up in 1970 by the Heath Government to examine the role of the nurse and the midwife in the hospital and the community (the Briggs Committee) is entitled the *Report of the Committee on Nursing*. Although the Committee stressed the difference in function between nurses and midwives, its recommendations for a joint regulatory body (albeit with a special Standing Committee on midwifery) have aggravated midwives' fears that they will henceforth be classed, officially as well as unofficially, with nurses, rather than as practitioners in their own right. Moreover, they question the wisdom of the Committee's proposal that all future midwives should also hold a nursing qualification, as they are already required to do in Northern Ireland and Scotland. This last proposal is, of course, in accord with the trend that has continued ever since the days of Mrs. Bedford Fenwick, and has been welcomed as an indication of the improved training and standing of the profession. However, the longer training and greater prestige of today's midwives make these concerns less relevant than they were seventy years ago. Furthermore, as nurses and midwives in training are increasingly treated more like students and less like cheap labour, the costs of their training will rise. The question is, therefore, whether Britain can afford to train a large number of workers for two jobs. 'Direct entry' midwives tend to stay longer in midwifery practice than do those holding a nursing qualification; some would therefore regard them as a 'better buy'.

Midwifery training itself may have to be extended before long. The Treaty of Rome calls for the harmonization of qualifications in member countries of the European Economic Community. For historical reasons, midwives in some of these countries enjoy a higher status than their English counterparts. French midwives, for example, are more highly educated and trained, and rank in the para-medical hierarchy as obstetric specialists on a par with dentists and chemists, rather than with nurses. Thus the Briggs Committee's proposals for a closer alignment of midwifery with nursing may prove not only expensive but inappropriate, being more suited to the needs of an earlier period than to the late twentieth century.

Let us now turn to child-bearing women themselves. Since the thirties the use of antibiotics has virtually eliminated puerperal fever, and, together with other obstetric advances, has cut maternal deaths in Britain to a tiny fraction of the pre-war figure. No longer, then, need British women fear the 'great dangers of Child-Birth'.[34] More attention, too, is being paid to the mother's emotional state during pregnancy and labour, and to the need to help her understand and co-operate in the birth process. To this end, some hospitals run classes to prepare mothers for childbirth and some (though by no means enough) allow husbands to be present to encourage and support their wives during labour.

Yet the system has its critics. Associated with the move to hospital delivery has been an increase in the incidence of forceps births, an increase in the use of episiotomy (cutting the perineum), and an increase in the proportion of births which are artificially induced. Predictably, these practices are seen in some quarters as efforts by the obstetrician to elevate and widen his role. It is, of course, the old question. Is the policy that all births should take place in hospital less in the interests of the patient than for convenience of the obstetrician? In Holland, it is pointed out, the majority of babies are born at home; yet maternal mortality (and perinatal mortality) are much lower than in Britain—indeed, among the lowest in the world. Again, is the man-midwife still too much for 'dispatch'? Are the benefits claimed for the large-scale use of episiotomy and induction great enough to outweigh the known disadvantages? Is the possibility of reducing the perinatal mortality rate by another decimal point worth subjecting growing numbers of women to the extreme pain often associated with induction, the resulting greater use of anaesthetics and the increased risk of the child's requiring intensive care?[35] Or is all this merely 'meddlesome midwifery'—modern style?

These and similar questions are currently being asked by the new organizations representing users of health services which have grown up in recent years as part of the general consumer movement.

Among these, the Patients' Association, the Association for the Improvement of Maternity Services (AIMS) and, a more recent arrival, the Society to Support Home Confinements, concern themselves with the quality of maternity care. The deliberate run-down of the domiciliary midwifery service, AIMS points out, denies the choice of home confinement to women who would prefer it; and as a recent survey has shown, over 80% of women interviewed who had experienced both home and hospital confinement preferred to have their babies at home.[36] Soon, however, the choice, and even the knowledge on which to base a choice, will no longer exist.

It is not only the articulate middle-class minority who question these developments. Medical opinion, as the present debate on induction indicates, is also divided,[37] and there are those who suggest that practices hotly defended as progressive today may tomorrow rank with wholesale tonsillectomy and other discredited medical fashions of the past. In this situation, as Cochrane and others have demonstrated, maternity services would benefit from the application of the rigorous tests of different methods of care now being mounted in other medical areas. At a time when hospital costs are rapidly rising, yet distressing gaps in our health services still remain, people are beginning to ask whether we should continue to accept arrangements which may perhaps prove of less benefit to the patient than to the medical profession.[38]

Another dimension has been added to the argument by the dynamism of the new Women's Liberation movement, which had its rise in the United States. Freed from the prudery which inhibited the early feminists, today's militants take pride in their female functions, and call for the right to choose how they exercise them. Along with demands for the abolition of the 'double standard' in sexual morality and for adequate contraception and abortion services, the movement is fighting for more sensitive health care for women—whose problems, whether physical or emotional, are, they claim, still not properly understood by a predominantly male medical profession.

In the United States the movement is campaigning against a system of maternity care which in most areas forces childbearing women into hospital to be delivered by men. It is a rejection of the dehumanizing, assembly line procedures of the institution, where, instead of being the central figure in a family drama, supported by husband and friends who can share in her great achievement, the woman is stripped of personal possessions and placed in stark, unfamiliar surroundings, to undergo among strangers what is usually a painful experience of at least several hours' duration, at the end of which her baby, the object of the exercise, may be whisked away to a communal nursery. The movement rejects routine episiotomy and anaesthesia (more common in the United States than in England), routine use of forceps, and the rack-like delivery bed on which the mother is strapped, flat on her back with her legs in stirrups, in a position which might have been deliberately designed to make her own efforts to bear her child as ineffectual as possible. In short, the women's protest is directed against procedures which they regard as part of a mystification of childbirth serving only the interests of the medical profession. It is also a protest against the male doctor's control over a basic female function—the pains—and joys—of which he can never experience nor fully understand, and which, it is alleged, he feels compelled to interfere with out of jealousy of women's generative powers.[39]

This rejection of the depersonalization of childbirth has led increasing numbers of American women to demand home delivery. Since few doctors are willing to give home attendance this has meant that many have sought the help of a midwife, in most States an illegal service. It was to meet the demand for home delivery in Santa Cruz (California) that in 1971 a number of women set up the Santa Cruz Birth Centre. So successful were Birth Centre midwives that by 1974 they were delivering 10% of all births in the Santa Cruz area. Predictably, the reaction of local medical men was hostile, and on their complaint prosecutions were set in train by the District Attorney. However, as a result of the consequent furor it is possible that Californian law may be revised to allow midwives to practise legally.[40]

Though the virtual disappearance of the American midwife is the result of over seventy years' effort directed to that end by the medical practitioners, there are some in the profession who have fought for the continuance of her work. Among these is the obstetrician Louis Hellman, Deputy Assistant Secretary for Population Affairs at the Department of Health, Education and Welfare,[41] who has long been a crusader for 'nurse-midwifery'. In New York, too, there has for some years been a small number of trained 'nurse-midwives' working in hospitals. However, these women were only allowed to assist the obstetrician at the birth, until in 1971 the College of Obstetricians and Gynaecologists finally consented to co-operate with midwives attending births independently. Immediately training programmes for midwives expanded,[42] and there was an enthusiastic demand for places.

At the same time, two other factors have brought the midwife before the public eye. One is the belated recognition that the United States' maternal mortality rate is higher than that of comparable European countries where midwives attend a majority of the births.

The other is the realization—equally belated—that the medical profession cannot efficiently undertake all obstetric care. This reappraisal of the situation has led to official acceptance of the part trained midwives could play in filling the serious gap which exists in the maldistributed American health services and in helping to reduce the high infant mortality rate.[43] Thus it may be that these pressures, coupled with the demands of 'Women's Lib' campaigners for giving choice to childbearing women, may at last bring back the midwife to the American scene.

Paradoxically, it appears that in Britain the revival of the feminist movement, and its success in gaining legislation to outlaw sex discrimination,[44] is likely to result in a restriction of female attendance in childbirth. Under the recent Sex Discrimination Act men are to be allowed to qualify as midwives. This development stems from the recent demands of a few male nurses for the right to enter the midwifery profession. Women, they protest, have no monopoly of understanding and care.[45] Men have been excluded from midwifery by a conservative body of women who have conspired to reserve it for the female sex—an accusation which, of course, takes no account of the medical profession's long-standing opposition to the establishment of a subordinate class of male practitioners. Ironically, these complaints would most probably have gone unheeded, were it not for the support they have received from some sections of the feminist movement who find it illogical to demand equal access to male-dominated occupations while men are excluded from the midwifery profession. Dismissing any objections as the product of an outmoded prudery, these women argue that what is sauce for the goose is sauce for the gander. After all, most doctors are men; why, then, should there be any objection to men acting as midwives?

Opponents of this view, who include the Royal College of Midwives, doubt if the majority of women, or their husbands, will welcome such a change.[46] Arguing that a midwife's sex is essential to her function, the College denies the analogy drawn between the proposed male midwife and the male obstetrician. The latter's relationship with the patient, the College points out, is of brief duration. In hospital, where most births now take place, he is chaperoned while carrying out any task of an intimate nature. This not only protects him from the temptation of taking sexual advantage of his patient, but also from the possibly greater risk that he might be accused of having done so. The work of a midwife, however, lasts over a longer period and is performed at regular intervals, often without the presence of another person. An increasing proportion of mothers are now discharged from hospital 48 hours after the birth, to be cared for during the post-natal stage in their own homes. It is during this period that the patient often seeks advice on the resumption of sexual relations and on family planning. In such circumstances, it was contended, a man would have considerable opportunity to take advantage of the patient, and would be correspondingly at risk from false accusations made by the unbalanced woman or the jealous husband. The appropriate analogy, therefore, was not with the obstetrician, but with the policewoman, the woman prison officer, or the woman customs official.

Indeed, the preponderance of men in obstetrics and gynaecology is seen by those opposed to the male midwife as an additional argument against admitting them to the midwifery profession. Most women, they maintain, feel more comfortable discussing matters relating to sex and reproduction with women rather than men. Yet, although a hundred years ago Parliament considered that a woman wishing to be attended by a female doctor should be able to have one, this choice is still not generally available in this country where less than a fifth of the medical profession are women. At a time when the need for the National Health Service to take greater account of the rights and preferences of patients is increasingly recognized, the College and its supporters pointed out that it was mothers and their babies for whom the midwife service was designed, and that in negotiating a deal to further the interests of their sex as workers, feminists should not be over-ready to trade in their interests as consumers.

However, it may be that, after all, few men will *want* to be midwives, and that the great majority of women who prefer a female midwife will be able to have one. More worrying, for those who value the mother's right to make such choices, is the officially encouraged policy of bringing all deliveries into hospital, and the increasing mechanization of labour which results. This has restricted the role of the (female) midwife and correspondingly widened that of the (usually male) obstetrician. Both these trends are now being hotly debated, not only in professional and feminist circles, but also by the wider public. But we have yet to see whether the new militancy of the women's movement will prompt British women to take the stand on home deliveries adopted by some of their American sisters and to espouse the midwife's cause.

Whatever happens, it is certain that the management of childbirth will never again be a female monopoly, and that the contribution of men over the last four centuries to obstetrics has made safe childbirth possible to a degree hitherto undreamed of. But until science discovers an alternative method of reproducing mankind, the predominantly male medical profession which now exercises so much control over pregnancy and parturition should not lose sight of the fact that it is women, and only women, who must carry and give birth to children, and that childbirth still remains, in the last analysis, 'women's business'.

Notes

CHAPTER 1   The Office of Midwife

1   C. J. Hyginus, *Fabularum Liber*, Basle, 1535, p. 63.

2   R. Barret, *A Companion for Midwives, Child Bearing Women and Nurses*, London, 1699, pp. 4–5.

3   J. Myrc, *Instructions to Parish Priests*, E. Peacock (ed.), London, 1902, lines 97–102.

4   J. McMath, M.D., *The Expert Mid-Wife and A Treatise of the Diseases of Women with Child and in Childbed*, Edinburgh, 1694, preface.

5   E. Ward, *The Whole Pleasures of Matrimony*, London, 1710, pp. 107–10; P. Willughby, *Observations in Midwifery. As Also the Countrey Midwifes Opusculum or Vade Mecum*, H. Blenkinsop (ed.), Warwick, 1863, p. 305; Barret, p. 7.

6   Willughby, pp. 11–12; see also the midwife's oath sworn by Ellen Perkins of St. Martin-in-the-Fields, London, in 1686 which bound her never to allow a woman to be delivered secretly, but always to see that the birth took place 'in the presence of two or three honest women, and that there be always two, or three lights ready if they may be had'. *Memorandum Book of Titus Wheatcroft*, 1722, p. 140, see Appendix 1.

7   T. Forbes (*The Midwife and the Witch*, New Haven, 1966, p. 149), quotes the Fabric Rolls of York Minster in an attempt to show that Agnes Hobson was 'presented' at the Bishop's Court in 1509 as an abortionist, and suggests that she was a midwife. In fact she was herself the victim of the abortionist—her master and lover, Richard Hall, a chaplain. See J. R. Raine (ed.), *The Fabric Rolls of York Minster*, Surtees Society, Newcastle, 1859, Vol. 35, p. 272.

8   R. Mannyng, *Handlyng Synne*, 1303, F. J. Furnivall (ed.), London, 1862, pp. 297–8.

9   Raine, p. 260.

10 A. Delacoux, *Biographie des Sage-Femmes Célèbres*, Paris, 1834, pp. 130–7.

11 J. Sprenger and H. Institoris, *Malleus Maleficarum*, trans. M. Summers, London, 1928, pp. 268, 66, 100, 140–1. See also M. Höfler, *Volksmedizin und Aberglaube in Oberbayerns Gegenwart und Vergangenheit*, Munich, 1888, p. 199.

12 W. Gubalke, *Hebammen im Wandel der Zeit*, Hanover, 1964, p. 16.

13 A. Fischer, *Geschichte des Deutschen Gesundtheitswesens*, Berlin, 1933, Vol. I, pp. 78–9; A. Querido, *The Development of Socio-Medical Care in the Netherlands*, London, 1968, pp. 15–16; H. Fasbender, *Geschichte der Geburtshülfe*, Jena, 1906, pp. 80–1.

14 E. C. J. von Siebold, *Versuch einer Geschichte der Geburtshülfe*, Berlin, 1839–45, trans. F. S. Hergott, as *Essai d'une Histoire de l'Obstetricie*, Paris, 1891–3, Vol. II, pp. 4, 30–40.

15 Fasbender, pp. 81–2.

16 'An Acte concernynge the approbation of phisycyons and surgions', *Public General Statutes of the Realm*, Henry VIII, 3, cap. 11.

17   J. Strype, *Annals of the Reign of Queen Mary*, London, 1706, p. 242.
18   Midwives' Letters Testimonial, *Guildhall Mss*, 10, 116. See Plate 1.
19   A. Boorde, *The Breviary of Helthe*, London, 1547, 'Extravagantes', fol. xvii.
20   Boorde, 'Extravagantes', fol. xvii; College of Physicians of London, *Annals*, III, 8 Sep. 1634, fol. 143b. R. S. Roberts, 'The Personnel and Practice of Medicine in Tudor and Stuart Times', *Medical History*, 6, 1962, pp. 363–4.
21   In 1662 the wife of William Silke (who was at the same time licensed as a surgeon) paid 13s. 6d. for her licence, plus other sums incidental to her application. *Canterbury Diocesan Archives*, LB 118 and LB 119 dorse. In Sterne's *Tristram Shandy* (set about ninety years later) Parson Yorick pays the fee of 18s. 4d. for Mrs. Wood the midwife. L. Sterne, *The Life and Opinions of Tristram Shandy, Gentleman*, London, 1760–7. Bk. I, Ch. VII.
22   Roberts, p. 368.
23   J. Guillemeau, *Child-birth or, the Happy Deliverie of Women*, London, 1612; W. Harvey, *Anatomical Exercitations, concerning the Generation of Living Creatures*, London, 1653.
24   Roesslin, *The byrthe of mankynd, otherwyse named the woman's boke*. Translated from the Latin by Thomas Raynalde, London, 1545, preface.
25   Roesslin, *The Byrth of Mankynde*, newly translated out of the Laten into Englysshe (by R. Jonas), London 1540, fol. VII (verso).
26   Louise Bourgeois, *Observations diverses sur la stérilité, perte de fruict, foecundité, accouchements, maladies des femmes, et des enfants nouveaux naiz*, Paris, 1617, Bk. II, pp. 104–5; Barret, pp. 1–2.
27   Willughby, pp. 2, 72.
28   Barret, p. 1.
29   Sarah Stone, *A Complete Practice of Midwifery*, London, 1737, p. xv.
30   Letter Testimonial relating to Mrs. Griffen, *Canterbury Diocesan Archives*, LB. 531.
31   Willughby, pp. 239, 73.
32   See Plate 1.
33   J. H. Aveling, *English Midwives: Their History and Prospects*, London, 1872, p. 34.
34   Bourgeois, 1617, Bk. II, pp. 104–5; Margaret Stephen, *The Domestic Midwife*, London, 1795, p. 62; W. M. Palmer, *Proc. Cambridgeshire Antiquarian Society*, 1911, p. 205; L. Sterne, *The Life and Opinions of Tristram Shandy, Gentleman*, London, 1760–7, Bk. I, Ch. VII.
35   N. H. Nicholas, *The Privy Purse Expences of Elizabeth of York*, London, 1830, p. 248.
36   *Calendar of State Papers, Domestic Series*, CLXVIII, 8 June 1630, p. 278.
37   Hester Shaw, *A Plaine Relation of my Sufferings by that Miserable Combustion*, London, 1653, pp. 1–2, 7, 11; *Mrs. Shaw's Innocency Restor'd*, London, 1653.
38   Anon., *The Midwives' Just Petition: or A Complaint of divers good Gentlewomen of that Faculty*, London, 1643.
39   N. H. Nicholas, *The Privy Purse Expences of King Henry the Eighth*, London, 1827, p. 197; G. N. Ormsby (ed.), *Selections from the Household Books of the Lord William Howard of Naworth Castle*, Newcastle, 1878, Surtees Society, Vol. 68, pp. 227–8, 263; R. Braybrooke (ed.), *Diary of Samuel Pepys*, London, 1893–9, Vol. I, pp. 203, 254; *Journal of the Reverend Giles Moore*, Sussex Archaeological Collection, Vol. I, p. 113.
40   Von Siebold, Vol. II, pp. 75–84.
41   The *Oxford English Dictionary* notes its use in 1625.
42   Von Siebold, Vol. II, p. 126.
43   Bourgeois, 1617, Bk. II, p. 235.
44   Willughby, p. 135.

45 See Plate 2.

46 This could happen to the most expert. In his *Treatise on Midwifery* William Smellie (1697–1763) relates how he once cut the umbilical cord too short, but passed it off to the midwife by pretending this was his method of preventing convulsions in the child. R. W. Johnstone, *William Smellie, the Master of British Midwifery*, Edinburgh, 1957, p. 204.

47 Harvey, pp. 488, 509.

48 Willughby, p. 6.

49 F. Mauriceau, *Des Maladies des femmes grosses et accouchées*, Paris, 1668, Bk. II, Ch. 8; H. Bracken, *The Midwives' Companion*, London, 1737, pp. 123–4; W. Clark, *The Province of Midwives in the Practice of their Art*, Bath, 1751, p. 16.

50 Willughby, pp. 248–9.

51 J. Graunt, *Natural and Political Observations, Mentioned in a following Index, and made upon the Bills of Mortality*, London, 1662, pp. 30–1.

52 ibid., p. 30. See also Harvey, p. 488; Jane Sharp, *The Midwives Book*, London, 1671, p. 3; McMath, preface.

53 Harvey, p. 488.

54 'The Thanksgiving of Women after Childbirth Commonly Called The Churching of Women', *Book of Common Prayer*, 1662.

55 College of Physicians, *Annals*, III, 3 June 1617, fols. 28b, 29a.

56 College of Physicians, *Annals*, III, 1617, fols. 28b, 29a; 1634, 141b, 143b, 144b, 145b; Report of the Enquiry into the Midwives' Petition, 22 Oct. 1634, quoted in J. H. Aveling, *The Chamberlens and the Midwifery Forceps*, London, 1883, pp. 46–7; Philalethes, *An Answer to Dr. Chamberlen's Scandalous and False Papers*, London, 1649, p. 2.

57 P. Chamberlen, *A Voice in Rhama: or, The Crie of Women and Children*, London, 1647.

58 Sharp, p. 182.

59 ibid., Preface addressed 'To the Midwives of England'.

60 *Observations diverses sur la stérilité, perte de fruict, foecundité, accouchements, maladies des femmes, et des enfants nouveaux naiz*, Paris, 1609. For an evaluation of this work, see Fasbender, pp. 156–9.

61 *Ein höchst nötiger Unterricht von schweren und unrechtstehenden Geburthen*, Coln an der Spree, 1690; see Fasbender, pp. 213–16.

62 Willughby, pp. 190, 201.

63 Nancy Mitford, *The Sun King*, London, 1966, Ch. VIII.

64 W. Sermon, *The Ladies Companion or, The English Midwife*, London, 1671, p. 5.

65 McMath, preface; Barret, pp. 3–4, Willughby, p. 157.

66 Sharp, pp. 2–4.

67 Willughby, p. 2.

68 Sharp, Preface: 'To the Midwives of England'.

69 Gubalke, p. 86.

70 The comment of Dorothy Osborne on the publication of a book of poems by the Duchess of Newcastle in 1653 illustrates this well. 'Sure, the poor woman is a little distracted, she could never be so ridiculous as to venture at writing books, and in verse too.' E. A. Parry (ed.), *The Letters of Dorothy Osborne to Sir William Temple, 1652–1654*, London, 1888, quoted in Myra Reynolds, *The Learned Lady in the Seventeenth Century, 1650–1760*, Boston, 1922, p. 51.

71 Fasbender, p. 145.

72 Henriette Carrier, *Origines de la Maternité de Paris*, Paris, 1888, pp. 81–3, 35–46.

73 Elizabeth Cellier, *To Dr . . .: An Answer to His Queries Concerning the Colledg of Midwives*, London, 1688.

74 Cellier, *A Scheme for the Foundation of a Royal Hospital*, Harleian Miscellany, London, 1745, Vol. 4.

75   Cellier, *To Dr . . .: An Answer to His Queries Concerning the Colledg of Midwives*.
76   Carrier, p. 90.
77   Fleetwood, J., *History of Medicine in Ireland*, Dublin, 1951, p. 139.
78   Helen Armet (ed.), *Extracts from the Records of the Burgh of Edinburgh, 1689 to 1701*, Edinburgh 1962, pp. 146–7.
79   Bourgeois, Bk. II, 1617, p. 215.
80   P. Dionis, *Traité général des accouchements*, Paris, 1718, pp. 444, 448, quoted in von Siebold, Vol. II, pp. 177–8.
81   Willughby, p. 135; J. Maubray, *The Female Physician*, London, 1724, p. 171.

CHAPTER 2   The Decline of the Midwife

1   Ivy Pinchbeck, *Women Workers and the Industrial Revolution, 1750–1850*, London, 1930, pp. 282–3, 304–6.
2   W. Radcliffe, *The Secret Instrument*, London, 1947, pp. 38–9.
3   Elizabeth Nihell, *A Treatise on the Art of Midwifery*, London, 1760, p. xii. John Page, a Lutterworth practitioner, writes of the 'credit' he gained after his first forceps delivery, and the resultant increase in his practice. E. Chapman, *A Treatise on the Improvement of Midwifery*, London, 1735, pp. 23–4.
4   Maubray, *The Female Physician*, p. 181; P. Thicknesse, *Man-Midwifery Analysed: and the Tendency of that Practice Detected and Exposed*, London, 1765, pp. 4, 22.
5   Nihell, p. 204; letter to the *London Gazetteer and Daily Advertiser*, June, 1772, Royal College of Surgeons Library.
6   The last midwife's licence appears to have been granted in the diocese of Peterborough in 1818. *Peterborough Diocesan Administrative Papers*.
7   Sterne, Bk. I, Ch. VII.
8   Jane Donegan, *Midwifery in America, 1760–1860*, Ph.D. thesis, Syracuse University, 1972, pp. 9–10.
9   *A Vindication of Man-Midwifery*, London, 1752, p. 6.
10   F. Nicholls, College of Physicians, *Annals*, 23 Mar. 1752; G. Counsell, *The Art of Midwifery*, London, 1752, p. xv.
11   Chapman, 1735, preface.
12   Stone, pp. x–xi, xvi, xix.
13   ibid., pp. xv–xvii.
14   Douglas, pp. 2, 66–7.
15   Dawkes, pp. 88–9.
16   Douglas, p. 47. The book was *Instruction Familière et très-simple, faite par questions et réponses touchant toutes les choses principales, qu'une sage-femme doit sçavoir pour l'Exercice de son art*, Paris, 1677. For an assessment of this work, see Fasbender, pp. 177–8.
17   Douglas, pp. 71–4.
18   R. Manningham, *The Institution and Oeconomy of the Charitable Infirmary for the Relief of Poor Women in Labour of Child and during their Lying-in*, London, 1739.
19   It has been suggested that Manningham's Infirmary later became Queen Charlotte's Hospital (G. C. Peachey, *Proc. R. Soc. Med.* (Epedemiology), 1924, 17, pp. 72–6) but a recently discovered contemporary publication disproves this. See *An Account of the Rise, Progress and State of the General Lying-in Hospital*, London, 1768, and Jean Donnison, 'Note on the Foundation of Queen Charlotte's Hospital', *Medical History*, 1971, pp. 398–400.
20   Carrier, pp. 48–9. The average number of patients delivered in the City of London Hospital between March 1750 and January 1827 was 383 p.a.; between 1749 and 1813 the British Lying-in Hospital averaged 487 patients p.a. (*Account of the City of London Lying-in Hospital, from March 1750–1 January 1827*, London, 1827; *Account of the British Lying-in Hospital*, London, 1814).

It is doubtful if either of the other two London lying-in hospitals exceeded these figures during this period.

21 *An Account of the Rise and Progress of the Lying-in Hospital for Married Women in Brownlow Street*, 1752; British Lying-in Hospital, *Minutes*, 9 Feb. 1787; *Account of the City of London Lying-in Hospital*, London, 1763.

22 See, for example, Marylebone Overseers of the Poor, *Accounts*, 24 April 1730, 'Paid Pitham to get a woman in Lab^r out of the Parish & Relived her 3s. 6d.'

23 See Hendon Overseers of the Poor, *Accounts*, 5 Jan. 1717, 'Paid the Man-Midwife for laying Elizabeth Williams, £3.4.6d.'

24 *An Account of the Rise and Progress of the Lying-in Hospital for Married Women in Brownlow Street*, London, 1752.

25 Nihell, pp. 44–5.

26 This could be as much as £30–£50 for a five to seven year apprenticeship. J. Collyer, *The Parent's and Guardian's Directory*, London, 1761, p. 196.

27 Sterne, Bk. I, Ch. VII.

28 Between 1754 and 1807 there are nine pupils recorded in this category, though these become less frequent towards the end of the period.

29 For a list of these outdoor medical charities in London and dates of foundation see A. B. Granville, *A Report of the Practice of Midwifery at the Westminster General Dispensary for 1818*, London, 1819, pp. 3–4. The Middlesex Hospital started an out-patient department in November 1785. St. Mary's Hospital, Manchester, founded 1790, also had such a department, and by 1793 so had the Westminster Lying-in Hospital. The Queen's Lying-in Hospital (previously the General Lying-in Hospital), had one at least by 1809, when existing records begin.

30 Lying-in Charity, *Minutes*, 25 July 1766; Westminster General Dispensary, *Minutes*, 6 June 1774.

31 On average the number delivered in the four Lying-in Hospitals was about 1,400 p.a. (A. B. Granville, *A Report of the Practice of Midwifery at the Westminster General Dispensary for 1818*, p. 16). Between 1767 and 1819 the Lying-in Charity alone averaged 4,000 cases a year (*Account of the Lying-in Charity*, London, 1820); the Benevolent Institution for the Sole Purpose of Delivering Poor Married Women in their own Habitations, another of the larger London midwifery charities, had over 1,100 patients p.a. between 1780 and 1814 (A. Highmore, *Pietas Londoniensis; The History, Design and Present State of the Various Public Charities in and near London*, London, 1814, p. 381). By 1818 the Westminster General Dispensary had averaged 656 p.a. since its institution in 1774 (Granville, *A Report on the Practice of Midwifery at the Westminster General Dispensary*, p. 19).

32 Maternal mortality in the practice of the Westminster General Dispensary for 1774–81 was 1 in 271 deliveries, whereas the rate in the lying-in hospitals was at least five times as much (R. Bland, *Some Calculations of the Number of Accidents or Deaths which happen in consequence of Parturition taken from the Midwifery Reports of the Westminster General Dispensary*, London, 1781, pp. 6–7; C. White, *A Treatise on the Management of Pregnant and Lying-in Women*, London, 1773, pp. 332–5).

33 *A Plain Account of the Advantages of the Lying-in Charity for Delivering Poor Married Women at their own Habitations*, London, 1767.

34 G. E. Mingay, *English Landed Society in the Eighteenth Century*, London, 1963, p. 243.

35 In the space of ten years (1741–51) Smellie took over 900 male pupils. Smellie, *The Theory and Practice of Midwifery*, London, 1752–64, p. v.

36 Thicknesse, *Man-Midwifery Analysed*, 1765, p. 4.

37 At the birth of at least three of her children she was attended by Mrs. Draper,

and Dr. William Hunter waited in an adjoining room in case he should be needed, but he was not summoned. 'An Obstetric Diary of William Hunter, 1762–1765', J. M. Stark (ed.), reprinted from the *Glasgow Medical Journal,* 1908, pp. 5, 10, 12.

38 Thicknesse, *Man-Midwifery Analysed,* 1765, p. 39. To 'touch' was to perform a vaginal examination for the signs of pregnancy.

39 Thicknesse, *A Letter to a Young Lady,* London, 1764, p. 11; F. Foster, *Thoughts on the Times but chiefly on the Profligacy of our Women,* London, 1779, pp. 4–5.

40 O. R. MacGregor, *Divorce in England,* London, 1957, p. 11.

41 Foster, pp. 6, 17–24, 31, 79.

42 Thicknesse, *Man-Midwifery Analysed,* p. 25; Foster, p. 196.

43 Thicknesse, *A Letter to a Young Lady,* 1764, p. 11; *Man-Midwifery Analysed,* 1765, pp. 10, 21.

44 Thicknesse, *Man-Midwifery Analysed,* 1765, p. 15.

45 Anon., *The Trial of a Cause between Richard Maddox, Gent., Plaintiff, and Dr. M . . .,* London, 1754.

46 Nihell, pp. 80–6.

47 Maubray, *The Female Physician,* pp. 181–2.

48 Quoted in H. R. Spencer, *The History of British Midwifery, from 1650–1800,* London, 1927, p. 73.

49 Stone, pp. xi–xii.

50 F. Nicholls, *A Petition of the Unborn Babes to the Censors of the Royal College of Physicians,* London, 1751, pp. 8–11.

51 Quoted in Spencer, p. 55.

52 College of Physicians, *Annals,* 23 Mar. 1752.

53 Nihell, pp. 44–9.

54 Thicknesse, *Man-Midwifery Analysed,* 1765, p. 28; Anon., *The Danger and Immodesty of the Present too General Custom of Unnecessarily Employing Men-Midwives in the Business of Midwifery,* London, 1772, Letter II.

55 Nihell, pp. 92–5; Thicknesse, *Man-Midwifery Analysed,* 1765, p. 22; *The Danger and Immodesty,* Letter II.

56 Nihell, pp. 158–9.

57 'Old Chiron', *Gazetteer and New Daily Advertiser,* 17 April 1772; L. Lapeyre, *An Enquiry into the Merits of these Two Important Questions . . .,* London, 1772, pp. 27, 35.

58 E. Chapman, *A Treatise on the Improvement of Midwifery,* London, 1753, preface.

59 Stephen, pp. 55, 107.

60 Martha Mears, *The Pupil of Nature,* London, 1797, p. 93.

61 Stephen, p. 105.

62 In his diary for 29 Mar. 1797, Parson Woodforde recorded that his apothecary, Mr. Thorne, had prescribed for his niece Nancy large quantities of port. 'She has not drank less than a Pint for many Days.' *Diary of a Country Parson,* J. Beresford (ed.), London, 1924–31, Vol. V, p. 22.

63 J. Adlard (ed.), *The Debt to Pleasure,* Cheadle, 1974, p. 92.

64 Ward, *The London Spy Compleat,* 1704, Vol. 2, pp. 396–9.

65 White, pp. 338–41.

66 Nihell, p. 70 (emphasis added). The Poor Law records for Marylebone and Islington bear this out. In 1731, Mrs. Fletcher, a Marylebone midwife, received 7s. 6d. (2s. 6d. more than the normal fee of 5s.) for 'an extraordinary case'. Marylebone Overseers of the Poor, *Accounts,* 19 Nov. 1731. However, where the man-midwife was called in to such cases, as he was in Islington, he received a guinea. Islington Overseers of the Poor, *Accounts,* 26 March 1756, 5 July 1756; 26 Aug. 1757.

67 Nihell, pp. xii, 28–36, 317–25.

68 ibid., pp. 217–18. The case of Elizabeth Blackwell, wife of Alexander Black-well, a Scots physician, illustrates this well. Mrs. Blackwell took up midwifery at her husband's suggestion in order to retrieve the family fortunes, but gave it up because she could not bear the low conditions in which she had to begin practice. Instead she compiled her *Curious Herbal* (1737) for which she is justly remembered.

69 ibid, p. 65.

70 ibid., p. 190.

71 Collyer, pp. 278–9.

72 Foster, p. 95.

73 *Gentleman's Magazine*, May 1772, p. 234.

74 Stephen, pp. 104–5.

75 ibid., pp. 55–63.

76 ibid., p. 62.

77 G. Crabbe, *The Parish Register*, 1807, Pt. III, in *Poems*, London, 1886.

78 ibid.

79 Nihell, p. 469; S. Fores ('John Blunt'), *Man-Midwifery Dissected*, London, 1793, p. 180.

80 Stephen, pp. 5–6, 20.

81 ibid., p. 4.

82 ibid., p. 43.

83 ibid., p. 19.

84 J. Hamilton, *A Letter to Sir William G. . . .*, Edinburgh, 1817.

85 The records of the British Lying-in Hospital show only sixty or so midwife pupils as having trained there during this period. Records of the City of London Lying-in Hospital and of the Westminster Lying-in Hospital do not contain this information, and those of Queen Charlotte's, which exist from 1809, indicate that only a handful were trained there during the following decades.

86 J. D. H. Widdess, *A History of the Royal College of Physicians of Ireland, 1654–1963*, Edinburgh, 1963, p. 198; T. P. Kirkpatrick, *The Book of the Rotunda Hospital*, London, 1913, pp. 98–9.

87 Fischer, Vol. II, pp. 60–1, 233–4.

88 J. Raulin, *Instructions Succinctes sur les Accouchemens en faveur des sages-femmes des provinces*, Paris, 1770, pp. iii–v.

89 Delacoux, pp. 71–2.

90 Carrier, pp. 237–59.

91 See Ch. 5, p. 99, below.

92 Nihell, pp. 217–18; Fores, pp. 182–7.

CHAPTER 3   The Ascendancy of Men

1 C. Wall, *The History of the Surgeons' Company, 1745–1800*, London, 1937, p. 54.

2 G. Clark, *A History of the College of Physicians*, Oxford, 1964–72, Vol. II, p. 588.

3 Quoted in *Nursing Times*, 4 Jan. 1947.

4 F. Bamford and the Duke of Wellington (eds.), *The Journal of Mrs. Arbuthnot, 1820–1832*, London, 1950, Vol. I, p. 245.

5 Wall, pp. 206–10; Company of Surgeons of London, *Minutes*, 22 Nov. 1797.

6 *Medical Times*, 1866, 2, p. 267.

7 College of Physicians, *Annals*, 10 May 1808.

8 College of Surgeons, *Minutes*, 9 Mar. 1808.

9 E. Harrison, *Remarks on the Ineffective State of the Practice of Physic in Great Britain*, London, 1806, pp. 32–7; *Observations on the Projected Bill for Restricting the*

Practice of Surgery and Midwifery, by a General Practitioner, London, c. 1816, pp. 5–7.

10 E. Harrison, *An Address delivered to the Lincolnshire Benevolent Medical Society*, London, 1810, Appendix, p. 103.

11 G. Clark, Vol. II, p. 632.

12 R. M. Kerrison, *An Inquiry into the Present State of the Medical Profession in England*, London, 1814, p. 27.

13 *Medical and Physical Journal*, Vol. 36, p. 284.

14 One of the earliest examples of its use is to be found in the *Medical and Physical Journal* in 1813, Vol. 29, p. 3.

15 Report of the General Committee of Associated Apothecaries, 13 November 1812, *Guildhall Mss*, 8299.

16 Associated Apothecaries, *Transactions*, London, Vol. 1, 1823, pp. xxxvi–xl.

17 A. B. Granville, *Autobiography*, Paulina Granville (ed.), London, 1874, 2, p. 212.

18 Parliamentary Committee of the College of Surgeons, *Minutes*, 26 June 1815.

19 Associated Apothecaries, pp. lix–lx.

20 *Lancet*, Vol. XII, pp. 460–1.

21 This was Robert Stott, successfully prosecuted by the Apothecaries' Society for unqualified practice as an apothecary. Society of Apothecaries Act of Parliament Committee, *Minutes*, 18 Oct. 1821; 17 May 1823.

22 *Lancet*, Vol. XI, p. 768.

23 Extract from a Memorial sent to Sir Robert Peel by the Obstetrical Society, probably early in 1828 (Royal College of Physicians Library).

24 Sir H. Halford to Sir R. Peel, March 1827, College of Physicians, *Annals*, 11 May 1827.

25 *The Times*, 18 May 1827.

26 Delacoux, passim.

27 Harriet Martineau writes of a Dr. Spencer in Bristol who trained his daughter as a midwife; such was the prejudice she encountered, however, that she became a governess instead. 'On Female Industry', *Edinburgh Review*, Apr. 1859, pp. 331–2.

28 Mary Wollstonecraft, *Vindication of the Rights of Women, with Strictures on Political and Moral Subjects*, London, 1792, pp. 192–3; Mildred Ellis, *The Education of Young Ladies of Small Pecuniary Resources for Other Occupations than that of Teaching*, London, 1838, p. 193.

29 *Lancet*, Vol. XII, pp. 205–6.

30 Granville, *A Report of the Practice of Midwifery at the Westminster General Dispensary for 1818*, London, 1819.

31 G. Jewell, *Lancet*, Vol. XI, p. 743.

32 S. Merriman, *Difficult Parturition*, London, 1820, p. 163.

33 *Medical and Physical Journal*, 1816, Vol. 35, p. 283 and n.

34 Anon., *Observations on the Impropriety of Men being Employed in the Business of Midwifery*, London, 1827, p. 45.

35 J. R. Pickmere, 'An Address to the Public on the Propriety of Women instead of Surgeons practising Midwifery', *Pamphleteer*, 1827, Vol. XXVIII, p. 67. *Observations on the Impropriety of Men being Employed in the Business of Midwifery*, pp. 26–48; *An Important Address to Wives and Mothers*, London, 1830, pp. 8–12; M. Adams, *Man-Midwifery Exposed*, London, 1830, pp. 1–83 (see page 234).

36 M. Adams, pp. 30–4, 63. A favourite target was a popular midwifery manual, *The London Practice of Midwifery*, which ran into several editions, the last being published in 1832. This manual recommended an accoucheur who was leaving a case in its early stages to introduce his finger into the patient's vagina, 'make a moderate degree of pressure', and then tell her that he had done something

which would be of great help to her in her labour. If all went well, he would then claim the credit, though absent. There was other similar advice on how to impress the patient, and the nurse, with his 'skill'. *The London Practice of Midwifery*, London, 1803 ed., pp. 139, 157–8.

37 *Lancet*, Vol. XII, pp. 118–19.
38 ibid., p. 457.
39 *The Principles and Practice of Obstetricy*, London, 1834, p. 213.
40 *Examiner*, 29 April 1827. Pickmere, p. 119; *Observations on the Impropriety of Men being Employed in the Business of Midwifery*, p. 45.
41 Highmore, pp. 202–3.
42 Society for Bettering the Condition and Increasing the Comforts of the Poor, *Extract of an Account of the Ladies' Committee for Promoting the Education and Employment of the Female Poor*, London, 1804, pp. 182–92.
43 The institution was directed by an ex-army surgeon, Dr. Walker Keighley. See British Ladies' Institution, *Address*, c. 1806.
44 See, for example, Priscilla Wakefield, *Reflections on the Present Condition of the Female Sex, with Suggestions for its Improvement*, London, 1796, pp. 131–9; Anon., *The Female Protector*, 1800. (Unpublished Ms., Fawcett Library.)
45 Pickmere, pp. 115–16; *Observations on the Impropriety of Men being Employed in the Business of Midwifery*, pp. 47–52.
46 Letter signed 'A', *Examiner*, 17 June 1827.
47 British Ladies' Lying-in Institution, *Prospectus*, in M. Adams, pp. 94–6 (see page 232). Later the charity was known as the Queen Adelaide's and British Ladies' Lying-in Institution.
48 At Queen Charlotte's this began in 1851, and at the City of London in 1862.
49 J. Adams, *Medical and Physical Journal*, Feb. 1816, pp. 87–8.
50 R. B. Cannings, *The City of London Hospital*, London, 1922, p. 25.
51 Registrar-General, *Annual Report* for 1841, pp. 185–6.
52 See *Returns from Her Majesty's Representatives Abroad of Laws and Regulations with reference to Midwives*, 1875, P.P. LXII, 255, 260, 268.
53 Charlotte Dall (ed.), *A Practical Illustration of Women's Right to Labour*, Boston, 1860, p. 56; Registrar-General, *Annual Report* for 1841, p. 186.
54 Registrar-General, *Annual Report* for 1841, p. 185.
55 ibid.
56 F. K. Brown, *Fathers of the Victorians*, Cambridge, 1966, pp. 438–9.
57 Bessie Rayner Parkes, *Remarks on the Education of Girls*, London, 1854, p. 11.
58 J. Brown and D. W. Forrest (eds.), *The Letters of Dr. John Brown*, London, 1907, p. 179.
59 *Lancet*, 1841–2, 2, Nov.–Feb.
60 ibid.
61 See *Lancet*, *Medical Times*, and *London Medical Gazette*, for 1844–5.
62 *London Medical Gazette*, 29 Aug. 1845, p. 782.
63 J. Struthers, *The Royal Colleges of Physicians and Surgeons under the Medical Act*, London, 1861, pp. 6–8.
64 R. M. Glover and J. B. Davidson, *The New Medical Act*, London, 1858, p. 45.
65 J. M. Kerr *et al.*, *Historical Review of British Obstetrics and Gynaecology, 1800–1950*, Edinburgh, 1954, pp. 296–8.
66 Obstet. Soc. Lond., *Trans.*, Vol. I, pp. v–xvi.
67 *British Medical Journal*, 1874, 1, p. 253.
68 *Lancet*, 1847, 2, p. 371.
69 ibid.
70 ibid., 1854, 1, p. 673; ibid., 2, p. 112.
71 In the Charity's Eastern district, 48,996 women were delivered in the years 1828–50 inclusive, with a rate of 4·5 per thousand dying within the month

after the birth. Only 3·3 of these deaths were due to puerperal causes. F. R. Ramsbotham, *Principles and Practice of Obstetric Medicine*, London, 1851, p. 718. In the Western district from 1852–64 inclusive the rate was 2·2 deaths per thousand deliveries. J. Hall Davis, *Parturition and Its Difficulties*, 1865, quoted in Kerr *et al.*, p. 263. The rate of maternal deaths per thousand *registered* births in England and Wales as recorded by the Registrar-General for the years 1847–54 inclusive was 5·4 and for the years 1855–64 inclusive was 4·75. ibid., p. 259.

72   *Lancet*, 1847, 2, p. 371.

73   See Ch. 4, p. 77.

74   In the 1841 Census only 743 women were recorded as midwives in England and Wales, though some may have been included among the 12,564 women returned as nurses. By the 1901 Census the figure had increased to 3,055, but this was clearly an underestimate, since when the Central Midwives Board first published the Roll in 1905, there were over 22,000 women enrolled.

75   See Jean Donnison, *The Development of the Profession of Midwife in England, 1750–1902*, Ph.D. thesis (Lond.), 1974, p. 109.

76   Queen Charlotte's Hospital, *Minutes*, 2 Nov. 1866.

77   Mrs. Mate, midwife to the Islington Union, who in 1847 and 1848 averaged 260 Poor Law cases a year, probably had at least £65 p.a. from this work alone. Islington Board of Guardians, *Minutes*, 13 Mar. 1849.

78   J. Browne, *The Accoucheur: A Letter to the Rev. Mr. Tattershall of Liverpool, on the Evils of Man-Midwifery*, London, 1859, pp. 15–16.

79   Select Committee on Medical Poor Relief, 1844, *Evidence; Report of Dr. E. Smith on the Metropolitan Infirmaries and Sick Wards*, P.P. 1866, LXI.

80   St. Mary's Hospital, Manchester, *Annual Report*, 1877. The figure for the Rotunda for the years 1851–3 inclusive was 17, 14 and 10 respectively. Select Committee on the Dublin Hospitals, *Report*, P.P. 1854, XII, App. 15, p. 349.

81   Harriet Martineau, 'On Female Industry', *Edinburgh Review*, April, 1851, pp. 331–2.

82   Mrs. Crewe, her epitaph tells us, 'during 40 years as a Midwife in this City brought into the world 9730 children'. F. Spiegel (ed.), *A Small Book of Grave Humour*, London, 1971.

CHAPTER 4   The Turn of the Tide

1   Pinchbeck, pp. 314–16.

2   *Journal of the Royal Statistical Society*, XLIX, March 1886, p. 321, Table II; and *Economic Development in the United Kingdom*, Labour Information, E.C.A. Mission to the United Kingdom, 1952, p. 218, quoted in the *Report of the Committee on One-Parent Families*, H.M.S.O., 1974, p. 35, Table 3.11.

3   H. Mayhew, quoted in W. Acton, *Prostitution Considered in its Moral, Social and Sanitary Aspects*, London, 1858, pp. 21–32.

4   *Westminster Review*, July 1850, pp. 448–506.

5   *Quarterly Review*, Dec. 1848, Vol. 84, pp. 179–80; *Fraser's Magazine*, Nov. 1844, Vol. 30, pp. 572–7.

6   ibid.

7   Wanda Neff, *Victorian Working Women*, London, 1966, pp. 165–71.

8   Governesses' Benevolent Institution, *Annual Reports* for the period.

9   Bessie Rayner Parkes, *Essays on Woman's Work*, London, 1865, pp. 55–6.

10   *Lancet*, 1857, 2, p. 229.

11   *Saturday Review*, 12 Nov. 1859, p. 576.

12   B. Abel-Smith, *A History of the Nursing Profession*, London, 1960, p. 5.

13   *Choice of a Business for Girls*, Tracts for Parents and Daughters, No. 3, London, 1864.

14 Abel-Smith, pp. 7–9.
15 Florence Nightingale, 'Cassandra', in Ray Strachey, *The Cause: A Short History of the Women's Movement in Great Britain*, London, 1928, pp. 395–418.
16 Abel-Smith, Ch. 1.
17 See J. Adams, op. cit., p. 87. 'A woman cannot always answer such calls [i.e. night calls] without some protection, which adds much to the difficulty and expence of her attendance.'
18 See *The London Practice of Midwifery*, pp. 138–9.
19 Quoted in Cecil Woodham-Smith, *Florence Nightingale*, London, 1951, p. 349.
20 Report on the King's College Hospital pupils, 15 July 1863, *Brit. Mus. Add. Mss.* 47714; 'Regulations for the Training of Midwifery Nurses under the Nightingale Fund', 18 Oct. 1861. *Nightingale Papers*, Greater London Record Office.
21 Florence Nightingale's comments on Dr. Sutherland's 'Notes on Midwifery Training', 27 June 1872, *Nightingale Papers*, Greater London Record Office; F.N. to Dr. H. W. Acland, 20 July 1869, 3 May 1873, *Nightingale Papers*, Bodleian Library.
22 ibid.
23 See Appendix 2.
24 J. Brown, *Horae Subsecivae*, Edinburgh, 1858, pp. xx–xxii.
25 *Lancet, Medical Times*, April–July 1850.
26 Browne, pp. iii–iv.
27 See *The Male Mid-Wife and the Female Doctor*, New York, 1974.
28 J. Stansfeld, 'Medical Women', *Nineteenth Century*, July 1877, p. 895.
29 Josephine Butler in a letter addressed 'Dear Friend' (probably Albert Rutson), 22 Feb. 1868, *Josephine Butler's Papers*, Fawcett Library.
30 Harriet Martineau, 'On Female Industry', *Edinburgh Review*, April 1859, pp. 331–2. Mrs. Isabel Thorne, one of the early medical students, and later the Secretary of the London School of Medicine for Women, considered she had lost a child because of the doctor's lack of interest in children's illnesses. E. Moberly Bell, *Storming the Citadel*, London, 1953, p. 69.
31 Josephine Butler, letter addressed 'Dear Friend'.
32 *Guardian*, 3 Nov. 1869.
33 *British Medical Journal*, 2 Aug. 1856, p. 653.
34 *Weekly Dispatch*, 11 Oct. 1857.
35 *Lancet*, 1858, 1, p. 44; ibid., 1861, 2, p. 117; ibid., 1865, 2, p. 435; ibid., 1868, 2, p. 644.
36 J. Hall Davis, *Parturition and its Difficulties*, London, 1865, p. 322.
37 *Lancet*, 1857, 2, p. 229; ibid., 1863, 1, p. 73, 2, p. 486; ibid., 1873, 2, p. 208.
38 Jo Manton, *Elizabeth Garrett Anderson*, 1966, Chs. IX–X.
39 *The Times*, 10 Oct. 1865.
40 See J. Edmunds, *Inaugural Address delivered for the Female Medical Society*, London, 1864.
41 See Elizabeth Blackwell, M.D., writing to her sister Dr. Emily Blackwell, in 1858, speak of 'the necessity of letting the midwife drop, and striving unflinchingly for the highest position'. *Pioneer Work in Opening the Medical Profession to Women*, London, 1895, p. 215.
42 *The Friend*, Tenth Month, 1865, adv. page; *Lancet*, 1866, 1, p. 720.
43 *Victoria Magazine*, Vol. 4, p. 282.
44 See B. Harrison, *Drink and the Victorians*, London, 1971, pp. 174–5. Two other supporters of the Female Medical Society, the Rev. Jabez Burns, and Archbishop Manning, were also active members of the temperance movement; see Appendix 4.
45 *Medical Times*, 1866, 2, p. 208. Dr. Edmunds drew this conclusion from the

1861 Census returns, which showed 5,000 or so medical men, but under 200 midwives, practising in London. Though this last figure was certainly an underestimate (see Ch. 3, p. 59 and note 74) the general conclusion was probably correct.

46   J. Edmunds, *The Times*, 10 Oct. 1865.

47   *Lancet*, 1866, 1, pp. 613–14; Edmunds, *Inaugural Address*, 1864.

48   *Medical Times*, 1866, 2, p. 208.

49   Edmunds, *Introductory Address, delivered . . . on the occasion of the opening of the Second Session of the Ladies' Medical College*, London, 1865.

50   *Lancet*, 1866, 1, p. 613.

51   *Victoria Magazine*, Vol. 8, p. 359.

52   *The Friend*, Tenth Month, 1865, adv. page; *Lancet*, 1866, 1, p. 613; *Victoria Magazine*, Vol. 8, p. 359.

53   *Lancet*, 1866, 1, p. 721.

54   ibid., 1865, 2, p. 435.

55   ibid., 1866, 1, pp. 613, 721; *The Times*, 26 June 1866; ibid., 26 May 1870.

56   Florence Nightingale, *Notes on Lying-in Institutions*, London, 1871, pp. 106–9. Florence Nightingale to Dr. Acland, 20 July 1869, *Nightingale Papers*, Bodleian Library.

57   Registrar-General, *Annual Report* for 1876, p. 250.

58   Obstet. Soc. Lond., *Trans.*, Vol. XI, pp. 132–4; Vol. XII, pp. 391–2.

59   Already in force in some Continental countries, this was not required here until 1927, and 1929 in Scotland.

60   Obstet. Soc. Lond., *Trans.*, Vol. XII, p. 402.

61   In 1874, however, the King's and Queen's College of Physicians of Ireland revived its earlier power to license midwives, but very few Englishwomen appear to have sought its diploma. See *British Medical Journal*, 1877, 1, p. 313.

62   Obstet. Soc. Lond., *Trans.*, Vol. XIV, pp. 21–3.

63   *Medical Times*, 1872, 1, p. 687.

64   Florence Nightingale to Dr. Sutherland, 23 Jan. 1872, *Nightingale Papers*, Greater London Record Office.

65   Aveling, *English Midwives*, pp. 169, 182.

66   Select Committee on the Protection of Infant Life, *Evidence*, QQ. 57, 791–809, 3760–1.

67   See *Medical Times*, 1868, 1, p. 222.

68   Aveling, *English Midwives*, p. 172.

69   Calculated on the basis of one midwife to 2,000 of the population of 23,000,000 in England and Wales. ibid., p. 171.

70   *British Medical Journal*, 1873, 1, p. 308.

71   Registration under this Act, compulsory on all wishing to dispense any drug officially scheduled as a 'poison', was open to all 'persons' (including women) already in business before 1 Aug. 1868 and to persons passing the officially approved examination of the Pharmaceutical Society.

72   *Medical Times*, 1873, 1, pp. 384–5.

73   James Stansfeld to Dr. Acland, General Medical Council, *Minutes*, 1873, Vol. X, p. 172.

74   *British Medical Journal*, 1873, 2, p. 677.

75   Obstetrical Association of Midwives, *Address . . . to All Women Practising Midwifery*, London, 1873.

76   National Association for the Promotion of Social Science, *Sessional Proceedings*, Vol. VII, pp. 285–7.

77   Aveling, *English Midwives*, p. 159.

78   Select Committee on Midwives' Registration, P.P. 1892, XIV, *Evidence*, QQ. 1359–60.

79 Dr. Elizabeth Garrett, *The Times*, 29 April 1870; Dr. Elizabeth Blackwell to Florence Nightingale, 30 Dec. 1871, *Nightingale Papers*, Greater London Record Office; *British Medical Journal*, 14 Oct. 1871, p. 455.

80 Dr. Blackwell to Florence Nightingale, 30 Dec. 1871.

81 A Lying-in Hospital for poor women, the 'Heidenreich von Siebold Stiftung', was founded in memory of her in Darmstadt where she practised. Gubalke, p. 93.

82 Anna von Helmholtz to Florence Nightingale, 7 May 1872; *Nightingale Papers*, Greater London Record Office.

83 *Scotsman*, 9 Mar. 1874.

84 *Lancet*, 1874, 2, p. 561; ibid., 1877, 1, p. 618.

85 ibid., 1874, 2, pp. 57, 561.

86 The Queen to the Princess Royal, 11 July 1860, quoted in R. Fulford (ed.), *Dearest Child*, London, 1964, p. 265.

87 *Lancet*, 1876, 1, p. 331.

88 *Scotsman*, 16 April 1876.

89 In the 1840s a few single women were working as out-door midwives for St. Mary's Hospital, Manchester, but these were daughters of midwives already on the staff. *Annual Report* of the Hospital for 1845-6.

90 Of the 87 'ladies' who had been through the Ladies' Medical College by May 1870, 46 were single women. *Victoria Magazine*, June 1870, p. 373. Out of 21 successful candidates in the Obstetrical Society's examination in April 1884, 19 were single. *Work and Leisure*, June 1885, p. 173.

CHAPTER 5 Midwives for the Poor

1 See *Englishwoman's Review*, Oct. 1873, pp. 277–8; also Jessie Boucherett, *The Condition of Working Women and the Factory Acts*, Helen Blackburn (ed.), London, 1896.

2 Obstet. Soc. Lond., *Trans.*, Vol. XVI, p. 26.

3 E. J. Tilt, *British Medical Journal*, 1874, 1, p. 288.

4 ibid, 1874, 1, p. 215.

5 G. Lord, *British Medical Journal*, 1873, 1, p. 354; *Medical Times*, 1873, 2, p. 609.

6 *British Medical Journal*, 1874, 1, p. 463.

7 ibid., 1874, 1, p. 252.

8 Charles Booth's survey of London, begun twelve or so years later, showed that one third of the population was living on or below a very stringent 'poverty line'. C. Booth, *Life and Labour of the People in London*, London, 1902. First Series, 'London Street by Street', p. 21.

9 G. C. T. Bartley, *The Seven Ages of A Village Pauper*, 1874, p. 54.

10 Royal Commission on Friendly and Benefit Building Societies, *Fourth Report*, P.P. 1874, XXIII, I, 143, 194, 205; Bartley, p. 106.

11 Charity Organisation Society, *Model Rules for Organising Provident Dispensaries*, London, 1878, pp. 12–13.

12 *British Medical Journal*, 1874, 1, pp. 252, 433.

13 G. C. T. Bartley, *The Poor Law and Its Effects on Thrift*, London, 1873, p. 15.

14 Dr. E. J. Tilt, *British Medical Journal*, 1873, 2, p. 676.

15 *Obstetrical Journal of Great Britain and Ireland*, Vol. I, p. 690.

16 *Lancet*, 1879, 1, pp. 746–7.

17 Thirty years later the percentage of births in voluntary lying-in wards in London (which was relatively well served in this respect) was thought to be between 5% and 6%, while throughout England and Wales the births in Poor Law Infirmaries were estimated at about 11,000, or a little over 1% of

total births. Royal Commission on the Poor Laws, *Minority Report*, 1909, pp. 78, 94.

18   Duncan, pp. 22-4.

19   J. Braxton Hicks to Florence Nightingale, 30 Jan. 1872, *Nightingale Papers*, Greater London Record Office.

20   Dr. Farr to Florence Nightingale, Feb. 1871. Dr. Rigden to Dr. Farr, 26 Jan., 30 Jan. 1871, *Nightingale Papers*, Brit. Mus. Add. Mss. 43400.

21   Nightingale, *Notes on Lying-in Institutions*, pp. 9-10.

22   Florence Nightingale to Dr. Farr, 27 Nov. 1871.

23   Obstet. Soc. Lond., *Trans.*, Vol. XVIII, pp. 90-272.

24   ibid., Vol. X, p. 86; *British Medical Journal*, 1885, 2, p. 1244.

25   Obstet. Soc. Lond., *Trans.*, Vol. XVII, pp. 130-5.

26   General Medical Council, *Minutes*, Vol. XII, pp. 133-7.

27   ibid., Vol. XIV, Appendix II, pp. 51-4.

28   General Medical Council, *Minutes*, Vol. XIV, pp. 195-6.

29   ibid.

30   *British Medical Journal*, 1878, 1, p. 438.

31   *Medical Times*, 1878, 1, pp. 446-7.

32   Obstet. Soc. Lond., *Trans.*, Vol. XXI, p. 6.

33   The Dentists Act followed the example of the Medical Act in the protection of registered titles and in not prohibiting unqualified practice, and of the Apothecaries Act, 1815, and the Pharmacy Act, 1868, in the admission to the register of all applicants already in 'bona fide' practice. However, applicants' qualifications were insufficiently checked by the G.M.C., and in the event many who were only apprentices and students and some who must have been only ten or eleven years old were admitted to the register. Inter-departmental Committee on the Dentists Act, 1878, P.P. 1919, XIII, *Report*, p. 7.

34   Obstet. Soc. Lond., *Trans.*, Vol. XXIII, p. 66.

35   Matrons' Aid Society Prospectus, c. 1881, *Brit. Mus. Add. Mss.* 47767.

36   In the eight years since the Society had instituted its examination, only 54 women had entered, 46 of whom were successful.

37   In the five years 1881-5, midwives trained in the British Lying-in Hospital, the General Lying-in Hospital, and Queen Charlotte's, numbered 49, 52 and 93 respectively, compared with 258, 218 and 633 monthly nurses. The first figures available for the City of London Lying-in Hospital relate to 1886, and show 16 midwives compared with 91 monthly nurses.

38   See E. A. Pratt, *A Woman's Work for Women*, London, 1898.

39   Emma Brierly, *Nursing Notes*, 1923, pp. 9-10.

40   *Pall Mall Gazette*, 9 Sep. 1880, p. 11.

41   *Work and Leisure*, Oct. 1880, p. 285.

42   Matrons' Aid Society Prospectus, *Brit. Mus. Add. Mss.* 47767. *Work and Leisure*, Feb. 1881, p. 37.

43   In 1884 the Islington Guardians' request for Local Government Board sanction to raise the fee paid to one of its midwives from 6s. to 9s., in consideration of the low income she had derived from the 101 Poor Law cases she had attended in her district in the preceding two years, was turned down. They were, however, allowed to pay 7s. 6d., a rate which was paid in only one other Union, and which the Board considered 'sufficient remuneration'. Islington Board of Guardians, *Minutes*, 24 Feb. 1884.

44   *Work and Leisure*, Mar. 1885, p. 65; *Englishwoman's Review*, 14 May 1887, p. 196.

45   Such was still the position twenty years later, and many busy midwives took three to four hundred cases a year in order to earn a living. Midwives' Institute, *The Midwife in Independent Practice Today*, London, 1936, p. 9.

46 Mme. Mourez, a brothel-keeper and abortionist who figured in the trial of W. T. Stead, was a midwife. G. Petrie, *A Singular Iniquity*, London, 1971, p. 251.
47 Matrons' Aid Society Prospectus, *Brit. Mus. Add. Mss.* 47767.
48 *Work and Leisure*, Mar. 1885, p. 65. Alice Gregory, daughter of the Dean of St. Paul's, who took up midwifery in the 1890s, wrote in her diary, 'I was one of the people God meant to take up the work.' E. Morland, *Alice and the Stork*, London, 1951, p. 31.
49 *Lancet*, 1882, 1, p. 508.
50 Matrons' Aid Society Prospectus and Regulations, *Brit. Mus. Add. Mss.* 47767.
51 Departmental Committee on the Midwives Act, 1902, P.P. 1909, XXXIII, *Evidence*, QQ. 2602–6.
52 Quoted Pratt, *A Woman's Work for Women*, pp. 88–9.
53 Marginal notes on the Matrons' Aid Society Prospectus, *Brit. Mus. Add. Mss.* 47767.
54 The Islington Guardians, who took reasonable care with their appointments, dismissed two successive midwives in 1892 and in 1893 for being drunk on duty. Islington Board of Guardians, *Minutes*, 28 April 1892; 30 June 1892; 26 June 1893. However, these were the only cases where drunkenness was mentioned in connection with the Board's midwives in the twenty years between 1880 and 1900. Flora Thompson's Mrs. Quinton, who practised at this time in rural Oxfordshire, was a 'sober, clean, intelligent woman'. *Lark Rise to Candleford*, Oxford, 1945, Ch. VIII.
55 *British Medical Journal*, 1882, 2, pp. 68–9.
56 *Medical Times*, 1882, 2, p. 91.
57 ibid., p. 90.
58 *Lancet*, 1882, 2, p. 1092.
59 *Englishwoman's Review*, 14 April 1883, pp. 164–5.
60 *British Medical Journal*, 1885, 1, pp. 617, 962.
61 In 1887 the Queen had devoted the bulk of the money collected by women as a gift to mark her Golden Jubilee (about £70,000) to the cause of district nursing.
62 *Nursing Notes*, 1923, p. 125.
63 An exception to the rule that pupils paid for training was the Jessop Hospital, Sheffield, where they trained for a year and were paid an annual salary of £9.
64 *Nursing Notes*, 1888, pp. 10–11.
65 On one occasion Miss Gregory called local mothers together to tell them that she proposed to raise her fee from 5s. to 8s. If they could not afford this, she told them, they should consider whether they had a right to bring the child into the world. Morland, p. 40.
66 See Ch. 7, pp. 141–2.
67 There were 325 midwives so employed in 1890. Dr. MacCabe, Irish Local Government Board, quoted by Dr. R. Rentoul, *British Medical Journal*, 1890, 2, p. 1174.
68 In 1911 perhaps a quarter of the Irish population received its ordinary medical care through the dispensary system. B. B. Gilbert, *The Evolution of National Insurance in Great Britain*, London, 1966, p. 398.
69 See Ch. 6, p. 124.
70 These were the Kensington, Crumpsall (Manchester) and Brownlow Hill (Liverpool) Infirmaries.
71 Margaret Llewellyn Davies (ed.), *Life as We Have Known it, by Co-operative Working Women*, London, 1931, pp. 42–6.
72 Queen Charlotte's Hospital described its objects in training midwives and monthly nurses in these terms.

73 H. Burdett, *Hospital Annual*, London, 1890, xcii. According to Charles Booth's London survey, monthly nurses seldom earned less than 21s. a week plus their keep during their engagements. *Life and Labour of the People in London*, Second Series, 'Industry', p. 95.

74 *British Medical Journal*, 1888, 2, p. 1060.

75 ibid., 1888, 2, p. 1132.

76 *Nursing Notes*, 1888, p. 89.

77 *Hospital Nursing Mirror*, 1 June 1889, p. xxxi.

78 *Nursing Record*, Vol. 1, p. 343.

79 ibid., 1888, 2, p. 378.

80 Mrs. Bedingfield, *Hospital Nursing Mirror*, 19 Oct. 1889, p. xv.

81 *British Medical Journal*, 1889, 2, p. 1370.

82 ibid., p. 1362.

83 *Lancet*, 1889, 2, p. 1176.

84 *Nursing Record*, Vol. 3, p. 330.

CHAPTER 6 Medical Men and Midwives Bills

 1 G. Webster, *Lancet*, 1852, 1, pp. 412–13.

 2 The Lying-in Hospitals were excluded.

 3 *Nursing Record*, Vol. 5, p. 98.

 4 Select Committee on Midwives' Registration, 1892, *Evidence*, Q.Q. 1305–6.

 5 The Liverpool Ladies Lying-in Charity had amalgamated in 1869 with the Liverpool Maternity Hospital, and there was no woman on the new Board.

 6 *Nursing Record*, Vol. 14, p. 416.

 7 *British Medical Journal*, 1890, 1, p. 682.

 8 *Hansard*, Third Series (Commons), Vol. 344, 21 May 1890, Cols. 1541–3.

 9 Mr. Hugh Owen, Secretary to the Local Government Board, to Sir Charles Lennox Peel, Clerk to the Privy Council, 7 July 1890. *Local Government Board Papers*, M.H. 19/188.

10 See *Provincial Medical Journal*, and *British Medical Journal*, 1890–1.

11 In 1893 the Islington Guardians asked its Medical Officers if they would undertake all the out-door Poor Law midwifery, and they 'unanimously' refused. Islington Board of Guardians, *Minutes*, 29 June 1893.

12 Select Committee on Midwives Registration, 1893, *Report*, Appendix I.

13 *Lancet*, 1891, 1, pp. 514–15.

14 J. de Styrap, *The Young Practitioner*, London, 1890, p. 392.

15 Dr. C. J. Cullingworth, Visiting Examiner for the Obstetrical Society, had found that often midwives knew more about the mechanism of labour than the average medical student. *Lancet*, 1890, 1, p. 1144.

16 See *Lancet, British Medical Journal*, 1890–1.

17 E. Arters, 'Midwife', *The Echo*, June 1890, quoted in *Nursing Notes*, July 1890 Supplement, p. 1.

18 Obstet. Soc. Lond., *Trans.*, 1891, Vol. XXXIII, p. 55.

19 On the 1879 Dentists' Register there were 5,289 persons, over 90% of whom were enrolled as 'bona fide' practitioners. Estimates of the number of midwives in practice varied from 7–20,000, supporters of registration putting it at 10–15,000. However, when the Roll was finally published in 1905 it was seen that even 20,000 had been an under-estimate.

20 Florence Nightingale continued sceptical on the supposed benefits of registration. At the time of the 1890 Bill, she had tried to impress upon Miss Paget her fears about the 'awful nature' of the Obstetrical Society's examination, the 'great want of training', and the problems likely to result from the large numbers of untrained women to be allowed on to the register as 'bona fide'

midwives. But Miss Paget, she complained, stuck to registration 'as a Panacea'. Florence Nightingale to the Queen Victoria Jubilee Nursing Institute, 19 June 1890, *Nightingale Papers*, Greater London Record Office.

21 *Lancet*, 1891, 1, pp. 55–6.
22 *Medical Press and Circular*, 26 Nov. 1890, p. 556.
23 *Nursing Record*, Vol. 6, pp. 98–9, 110.
24 Select Committee on Midwives' Registration, 1892, 1893, *Evidence*.
25 All the Act did, however, was to require that all *registered medical practitioners* should be qualified in medicine, surgery, and midwifery.
26 Of the 150 or so women on the Medical Register, about 20 practised in London, one or two in each of the large provincial towns, while the rest (roughly four-fifths) were in India.
27 Select Committee on Midwives' Registration, 1893, *Report*.
28 *British Medical Journal*, 1891, 1, p. 230.
29 Queen Charlotte's Hospital and the General Lying-in Hospital had both been particularly unfortunate with persistent outbreaks of puerperal fever, but with the 'careful use of antiseptics' the maternal death-rate had been greatly reduced in both hospitals.
30 Obstet. Soc. Lond., *Trans.*, 1885, Vol. XXVII, p. 218.
31 *Nursing Record*, Vol. 10, p. 302.
32 *Provincial Medical Journal*, Oct. 1893, p. 539.
33 General Medical Council, *Minutes*, 1892, Vol. XXIX, p. 112.
34 *British Medical Journal*, 1894, 1, pp. 435–6.
35 ibid., 1890, 1, p. 682.
36 See E. M. Little, *History of the British Medical Association, 1832–1932*, London, 1932, pp. 79–87.

Chapter 7 State Register or Local Licence?
1 B. L. Hutchins and A. Harrison, *A History of Factory Legislation*, London, 1926, p. 210.
2 The Women's Co-operative Guild was founded in 1883; the (Conservative) Primrose League in 1885; the Women's Liberal Unionist Association and the Women's Liberal Federation in 1886.
3 Although the word 'compulsory' appeared in the Association's title it was in fact against *compulsory* registration and opposed the prohibition of practice by the unqualified woman. See p. 149 below.
4 A.P.C.R.M., Report for 1900–1, Home Office Papers HO/45/10129.
5 *Nursing Record*, Vol. 12, p. 354; Vol. 13, pp. 105, 394. Though Mrs. Fenwick's prophecy was largely fulfilled, even today about one eighth of practising midwives have neither general nursing nor sick children's nursing qualifications.
6 *Nursing Record*, Vol. 13, p. 166.
7 *Nursing Notes*, 1895, pp. 57–9.
8 *British Medical Journal*, 1895, 1, pp. 1120–1.
9 *Lancet*, 1895, 1, p. 1258; *Hospital*, Vol. 18, pp. 107–8, 181.
10 *British Medical Journal*, 1895, 1, pp. 1281–2.
11 *Nursing Record*, Vol. 14, pp. 97–8, 177.
12 *British Medical Journal*, 1896, 1, p. 1048.
13 See *Nursing Record*, Vol. 17, pp. 181–2, 201–2.
14 *British Medical Journal*, 1895, 2, pp. 219–21; 1896, 1, pp. 372–4; *Lancet*, 1896, 1, p. 1310.
15 *Medical Times and Hospital Gazette*, 4 July 1896, p. 421; *Nursing Record*, Vol. 16, p. 128.
16 Dr. W. M. Banks, *British Medical Journal*, 1896, 2, p. 43.

17   Lady Priestley, 'Nurses à la Mode', *Nineteenth Century*, 1896, p. 29.

18   *Nursing Record*, Vol. 16, pp. 349–50.

19   Morland, p. 34.

20   Queen's Nursing Institute Council, *Annual Reports*, 1896, 1897. These women had also to possess an approved certificate in midwifery.

21   E. Pratt, *Pioneer Women in Victoria's Reign*, pp. 153–8. Miss Twining was cousin to Miss Louisa Twining, the workhouse reformer.

22   The usual charge of the Mortlake Nursing Association was 7s. 6d., but where the husband earned 30s. it was 10s. *British Medical Journal*, 1896, 2, pp. 1523, 1679.

23   Morland, p. 43.

24   *British Medical Journal*, 1896, 2, p. 1523.

25   *Nursing Record*, Vol. 16, p. 490.

26   The Prussian district midwife whose training had been paid for by the community had to work for at least three years in a district post, and keep a case-book for inspection by the Medical Inspector. Both she and the midwife in private practice had to submit themselves to three-yearly examinations by the Inspector on the extent of her knowledge. *Returns from Her Majesty's Representatives abroad of Laws and Regulations with Reference to Midwives*, P.P. 1875, LXII, 269–71.

27   The actual words were: 'For disobeying the rules and regulations from time to time laid down under the Act by the Midwives Board or for other misconduct.'

28   See Ch. 9, p. 183 below.

29   *Nursing Notes*, 1897, p. 92.

30   *Lancet*, 1897, 1, pp. 156–7.

31   ibid., 1896, 1, p. 1144; *Nursing Notes*, 1897, p. 20.

32   R. R. Rentoul, *A Draft Bill to provide for the Compulsory Registration and Supervision of Midwifery and Other Nurses*, London, 1897.

33   *British Medical Journal*, 1898, 1, p. 574.

34   C. J. Cullingworth, M.D., 'The Registration of Midwives', *Contemporary Review*, March 1898, pp. 394–5.

35   *British Medical Journal*, 1898, 1, p. 520. Horsley himself had for some time maintained that Section 40 of the Medical Act, 1858, could in fact be construed as forbidding unqualified practice (despite a clear statement to the contrary in the Act's preamble). The unsuccessful prosecution of Joseph Steel by the G.M.C. in 1898 proved that Horsley was wrong, and that it was only possible to get convictions against unqualified practitioners under the Apothecaries' Act, in which case they must be convicted of acting as an apothecary, i.e. of prescribing *and* dispensing.

36   *British Medical Journal*, 1898, 1, p. 575.

37   *Public Health*, 1898, p. 249.

38   *Lancet*, 1898, 1, p. 791.

39   Dr. Mary Scharlieb and Dr. Annie McCall.

40   *The Times*, 30 April 1898, p. 1269.

41   General Medical Council, *Minutes*, Vol. XXXV, pp. 22–5.

42   General Medical Council, *Minutes*, Vol. XXXV, p. 489; *Lancet*, 1898, 1, p. 1662.

43   *British Medical Journal*, 1898, 1, p. 1027.

44   *The Times*, 3 May 1898.

45   *Woman's Signal*, 1898, pp. 249, 286.

46   General Medical Council, *Minutes*, Vol. XXXV, pp. 503, 506.

47   Association for Promoting the Compulsory Registration of Midwives, Annual Report, 1897–8, *Nursing Notes*, 1898, pp. 91–4.

48 *Lancet*, 1898, 1, p. 1269.
49 General Medical Council, *Minutes*, Vol. XXXV, pp. 478–83.
50 *Nursing Notes*, 1899, p. 24.
51 *Nursing Record*, Vol. 22, p. 34.
52 ibid., pp. 34–5, 53.
53 ibid., p. 63.
54 Manchester Midwives' Society, *Transactions*, 1897–8, Manchester, 1899, pp. 41–65.
55 *Lancet*, 1897, 1, p. 546.
56 *British Medical Journal*, 1899, 1, pp. 350–3.
57 ibid., p. 349.
58 *Nursing Notes*, 1900, pp. 64–5.
59 *Nursing Record*, Vol. 23, p. 386.
60 The 'safeguards' were that final decisions in disciplinary matters should lie not with the local authorities, but with the Central Board, on which the representation of the Midwives' Institute and of the Privy Council should be retained. Existing midwives holding the certificate of the Obstetrical Society should automatically be admitted to the Roll without having to produce a certificate of good character.
61 *Nursing Notes*, July 1899, p. 101.
62 *Hospital*, Vol. 25, p. 46.
63 *British Medical Journal*, 1900, 1, pp. 279, 420–1.
64 *Lancet*, 1900, 1, pp. 549, 784.
65 *Hansard*, 4th Series (Commons), Vol. 80, 9 Mar. 1900, Cols. 537–44.
66 *British Medical Journal*, 1900, 1, pp. 545–6, 653–64, 795, 878.
67 *General Practitioner*, 14 April 1900, p. 233; *Medical Times and Hospital Gazette*, 5 May 1900, p. 277.
68 *Practitioner*, pp. 361–2, 483.
69 *British Medical Journal*, 1900, 1, p. 1302.
70 ibid.
71 *Home Office Papers*, H.O. 45/10129.
72 *Nursing Notes*, 1900, pp. 110–11.
73 *Nursing Notes*, 1900, p. 111.
74 *Englishwoman's Review*, 17 April 1900, p. 118.
75 See *Returns on the Law relating to Still-births in England and Other Countries*, P.P. 1893–4, LXXIII, 355. The primary object of most American midwife legislation was to control and limit midwife practice rather than to improve her training and status. New York Academy of Medicine, *Maternal Mortality in New York City*, New York, 1932, p. 191. By 1918 midwife practice in Massachusetts had been made illegal, as it now is in most States of the Union.
76 *Lancet*, 1900, 1, p. 872.

CHAPTER 8   The Midwives Act, 1902

1 For the development of the controversy see *British Medical Journal, Lancet, General Practitioner, Medical Times and Hospital Gazette*, 1901–2.
2 See *Nursing Notes*, Dec. 1901–Feb. 1902.
3 *The Times*, 24 Dec. 1901.
4 *Hospital*, Vol 31, p. 231.
5 These certainly included Lord Balfour of Burleigh, who had been in charge of the 1895 Bill, and probably the Earl of Selborne and Sir Michael Hicks-Beach, whose wives were both active workers for registration. Mr. C. T. Ritchie, Home Secretary, was also well disposed towards the Bill. *British Medical Journal*, 7 June 1902, pp. 1427, 1438–40.

6 *Nursing Notes*, 1901, p. 141.
7 *Hansard*, Fourth Series (Commons), Vol. 103, Col. 1157.
8 *British Medical Journal*, 1900, 1, p. 797.
9 *Home Office Papers*, H.O. 45/10129, 20 Mar. 1902.
10 *Nursing Record*, Vol. 28, pp. 142, 179.
11 *Nursing Notes*, 1902, p. 95; *Hansard*, Fifth Series (Commons), Vol. 311, Col. 1198.
12 For the debate on the Bill see *Hansard*, Fourth Series (Commons), Vol. 103, Cols. 1152–1211.
13 *British Medical Journal*, 1902, 1, pp. 675–8, 723–35.
14 *Nurses' Journal*, April 1902, p. 52.
15 *Nursing Notes*, 1902, p. 86.
16 *Nursing Notes*, 1902, pp. 70–1.
17 *British Medical Journal*, 1902, 1, p. 1056; *Lancet*, 1902, 1, pp. 607, 682–3.
18 *Medical Press and Circular*, 1899, 2, p. 93.
19 *Practitioner*, April 1902, pp. 369–71.
20 *British Medical Journal*, 1902, 1, p. 1451.
21 *British Medical Journal*, 1902, 1, pp. 1427, 1440.
22 ibid., 1902, p. 1237.
23 *British Medical Journal*, 1902, 1, p. 1491.
24 *Nursing Notes*, 1902, p. 141.
25 ibid., pp. 114–15.
26 There are now practically no midwives practising in Canada. See International Federation of Gynaecology and Obstetrics and the International Federation of Midwives, *Maternity Care in the World*, Oxford, 1966, p. 128. In the United States in 1964 midwives (mostly untrained 'Granny midwives' practising amongst the poor coloured population in rural areas) attended about 1·5% of births. A few trained nurse-midwives worked for the Frontier Nursing Service in Kentucky and the Catholic Maternity Society in Santa Fe. S. Shapiro *et al.*, *Infant Peri-Natal, Maternal and Child Mortality in the United States*, Cambridge (Mass.), 1968, p. 258. See however Ch. 9, pp. 197–9.

CHAPTER 9 Conclusions

1 *Nursing Notes*, 1900, p. 35; 1902, pp. 110, 141.
2 General Medical Council, *Minutes*, Vol. XXXIX, p. 104.
3 *Lancet*, 1903, 2, pp. 616–17; *Nursing Notes*, 1903, pp. 91–3.
4 General Medical Council, *Minutes*, Vol. XLIII, pp. 200, 417.
5 The Dentists' Act, 1921, and the Veterinary Surgeons Acts of 1948 and 1966.
6 In 1916 training for candidates without nurse training was increased to six months. In 1926 this became a year, and in 1938 two years, with one year for State registered nurses. From January 1939, all practising midwives were required to go on a refresher course of at least four weeks once every seven years.
7 *Poor Law Officers' Journal*, 21 April 1905, 23 Mar. 1906.
8 One was suspended for three months; *Nursing Notes*, 1908, p. 243. Dr. H. Hanford, M.O.H. for Nottinghamshire, defended this practice to the 1909 Departmental Committee in the Midwives Act, *Report*, Q.Q. 4034–44.
9 Under the title, 'An Immoral Midwife', the Journal expressed its concern that an 'unchaste' and immoral midwife might corrupt both husband and wife. *Nursing Notes*, 1915, pp. 139, 150.
10 Similar powers were conferred on the General Nursing Council, set up in 1919. Eve Bendall and Elizabeth Raybould, *A History of the General Nursing Council for England and Wales, 1919–1969*, London, 1969, p. 114.

11 Only a State-registered nurse or a State-certified midwife might thereafter legally act as a maternity nurse.

12 *Nursing Notes*, 1913, p. 337.

13 Departmental Committee on the Midwives Act 1902, *Report*, 1909, p. 4; Ministry of Health, *Report of Departmental Committee on Maternal Mortality and Morbidity*, 1930, p. 105.

14 *Nursing Notes*, 1919, p. 37.

15 *Report on an Investigation into Maternal Mortality*, p. 253.

16 *Report on Maternal Mortality in Wales*, pp. 32–3.

17 Registrar-General's Statistical Review for 1937, quoted Kerr *et al.*, p. 340.

18 Ministry of Health, *Report of the Departmental Committee on the Training and Employment of Midwives*, 1929, p. 36.

19 Improved accuracy in death certification of later years may have resulted in more cases being attributed to maternal causes than earlier in the period and thus to a very slight rise in the recorded death rate. Another factor which may have produced a very small rise in the rate was the increased proportion of first births (always more dangerous than subsequent ones, up to the ninth) which was the result of the falling birth-rate, but this is likely to have been more than cancelled out by the accompanying decrease in high order births. For a discussion of these issues see Ministry of Health, *Report on an Investigation into Maternal Mortality*, 1937, pp. 41–63, 107–9, 302.

20 *Report on an Investigation into Maternal Mortality*, 1937, p. 20.

21 *Hansard*, 5th Series, Vol. 311 (Commons), Cols. 1117–19, 1160. Examples given by Sir Kingsley were the maternity charities in West Ham, a poor area in the East End of London, and the Queen's Nursing Institute, whose midwives worked in rural areas, delivering approximately 60,000 women a year.

22 Ministry of Health, 'High Maternal Mortality in Certain Areas', *Reports on Public Health and Medical Subjects*, pp. 60–69, 1932, 80–1.

23 J. S. Fairbairn quoted in J. M. Munro Kerr, *Maternal Mortality and Morbidity*, Edinburgh, 1933, p. 247.

24 *Report on an Investigation into Maternal Mortality*, pp. 283–4.

25 Ministry of Health, *Interim Report on Maternal Mortality and Morbidity*, 1930, p. 27.

26 Ministry of Health, *Final Report on Maternal Mortality and Morbidity*, 1932, p. 37.

27 Those who were compulsorily retired received compensation equivalent to five years' earnings and those who retired voluntarily a sum equivalent to three years' earnings.

28 In 1934 Dr. Minnit perfected his apparatus for the administration of nitrous oxide gas and air, which was approved by the Central Midwives Board for use by suitably trained midwives.

29 *Report of the Departmental Committee on the Midwives Act, 1902*, p. 2.

30 J. H. Turnbull, 'Note on the Observations of the Central Midwives Board on the Report of the Departmental Committee on the Training and Employment of Midwives', 4 Dec. 1929, *Ministry of Health Papers*, M.H. 55.

31 A note of reservation was signed by Dr. J. S. Fairbarn and Mrs. Bruce Richmond, both members of the Board, *Report of the Departmental Committee on the Training and Employment of Midwives*, pp. 84–8.

32 Minute by A. B. Maclachlan, 4 Dec. 1929, *Ministry of Health Papers*, M.H. 55.

33 See, however, p. 195 below.

34 The rate for England and Wales in 1975 was ·13 per 1,000 total births. *Office of Population Censuses and Surveys Monitor*, 1975/26.

35 See Sheila Kitzinger, *Some Women's Experiences of Induced Labour*, National Childbirth Trust, 1975.

36 AIMS, *Quarterly Newsletter*, March 1975, p. 7.
37 See *The Times*, 12 Aug. 1974.
38 A. L. Cochrane, *Effectiveness and Efficiency: Random Reflections on Health Services*, London, 1971, pp. 63–6.
39 Doris B. Haire, *Cultural Differences in Maternity Care* (Address to the Third International Congress of Psychosomatic Medicine in Obstetrics and Gynaecology, 3 Mar. 1971); The Boston Women's Health Book Collective, *Our Bodies, Ourselves: A Book By and For Women*, New York, 1971, pp. 182–205, 239–40.
40 *The San Francisco Bay Guardian*, 20 July 1974.
41 At the time of writing (1976).
42 Shirley Streshinsky, 'Are you Safer with a Midwife?', *Ms. Magazine*, Oct. 1973.
43 ibid.; *Los Angeles Times*, 25 July 1971; *The Sun*, 2 Nov. 1972; *San Francisco Bay*
44 *Guardian*, 20 July 1974.
45 *Sex Discrimination Act*, 1975.
   Guardian, 20 Feb. 1974.
46 Royal College of Midwives, *Sex Discrimination Bill—Male Midwives*, London, 1975.

Selected Bibliography

This bibliography lists some of the more important and readily available sources which will interest students of the history presented in this book. A much more extensive bibliography can be found in the thesis on which the book is based, *The Development of the Profession of Midwife in England 1750–1902*, available from the libraries of the University of London and the London School of Economics and Political Science.

Abel-Smith, B., *A History of the Nursing Profession*, London, 1960.

Acton, W., M.D., *Prostitution Considered in its Moral, Social and Sanitary Aspects in London and other large Cities & Garrison Towns*, London, 1857.

Adams, M., *Man-Midwifery Exposed . . . with broad hints to new married people, and young men and women*, London, 1830.

Atkinson, S. B., M.D., *The Office of Midwife*, London, 1907.

Aveling, J. H. M.D., *The Chamberlens and the Midwifery Forceps*, London, 1883.

—— *English Midwives: Their History and Prospects*, London, 1872.

Barret, R., *A Companion for Midwives, Child bearing Women, and Nurses, directing them how to perform their respective Offices*, London, 1699.

Bartley, G. C. T., *The Seven Ages of a Village Pauper*, London, 1874.

—— *The Poor Law and its Effects on Thrift, with suggestions for an improved out-door relief*, London, 1873.

Bell, Enid H. C. Moberly, *Storming the Citadel: The Rise of the Woman Doctor*, London, 1953.

Bendall, Eve and Raybould, Elizabeth, *A History of the General Nursing Council for England and Wales, 1919–1969*, London, 1969.

Blackwell, Elizabeth, M.D., *Pioneer Work in opening the Medical Profession to Women: autobiographical sketches*, London, 1895.

Bland, R., *Some Calculations of the Number of Accidents or Deaths which happen in consequence of Parturition etc. taken from the Midwifery Reports of the Westminster General Dispensary*, London, 1781.

Boston Women's Health Book Collective, The, *Our Bodies, Ourselves. A Book By and For Women*, New York, 1971.

Boucherett, Jessie, *The Condition of Working Women and the Factory Acts*, London, 1896.

Bourgeois, Louise, *Observations diverses sur la stérilité, perte de fruict, foecundité, accouchements, maladies des femmes et des enfants nouveaux naiz*, Paris, 1609, 1617;

Translated: *The Complete Midwife's Practice Enlarged . . . The Second edition corrected by R.C., I.D., M.S., T.B., Practitioners of the said art with a full supply of those rare secrets which Mr. Culpepper in his brief treatise of midwifery, & other English writers have . . . omitted*, London, 1659.

Bracken, H., *The Midwife's Companion, or, a Treatise of Midwifery*, London, 1737.

British Lying-in Hospital, *An Account of the Rise and Progress of the Lying-in Hospital for Married Women in Brownlow Street, London, from its first institution in November 1749 to July 25th 1751*. London, 1752, and later editions.

Cannings, R. B., *A Short History of the City of London Maternity Hospital*, London, 1922.

Carrier, Henriette, *Origines de la Maternité de Paris*, Paris, 1888.

Cellier, Elizabeth, *To Dr. . . .: An Answer to His Queries concerning the Colledg of Midwives*, London, 1688.

—— *A Scheme for the Foundation of a Royal Hospital, & raising a revenue of five or six-thousand pounds a year, by, & for the maintenance of a corporation of skilful midwives, and such foundlings or exposed children as shall be admitted therein*, London, 1745.

Chamberlen, P., M.D., *A Voice in Rhama: or the Crie of Women and Children*, London, 1647.

Chapman, E., *Essay on the Improvement of Midwifery; chiefly with regard to the operation*, London, 1733.

Cobbett, W., *Advice to Young Men (and Incidentally to Young Women) in the Middle and Higher Ranks of Life*, London, 1829.

Cook, E. T., *The Life of Florence Nightingale*, 2 vols., London, 1913–14.

Counsell, G., *The Art of Midwifry: or, the Midwife's sure guide: wherein the most successful methods of practice are laid down, in the plainest, clearest, and shortest manner*, London, 1752.

Crabbe, G., 'The Parish Register', 1807, in *Poems*, London, 1886.

Cullingworth, C. J., M.D., 'The Registration of Midwives', *Contemporary Review*, March, 1898.

Dall, Charlotte (ed.), *Woman's Right to Labor, or Low wages and hard work*, Boston, 1860.

Danger (The) & Immodesty of the Present too General Custom of Unnecessarily Employing Men-Midwives, London, 1772.

Delacoux, A., *Biographie des Sage-Femmes Célèbres, anciennes, modernes et contemporaines*, Paris, 1834.

Fasbender, H., *Geschichte der Geburtshülfe*, Jena, 1906.

Female Medical Society, *Inaugural Address delivered for the Female Medical Society on October 2, 1865, at the Hanover Square Rooms, by Dr. James Edmunds, upon the occasion of the opening of the second session of the Ladies' Medical College*, London, 1865.

Fischer, A., *Geschichte des deutschen Gesundheitswesens. . . . Herausgegeben von Arbeitsgemeinschaft sozialhygienischer Reichsfachverbande*, 2 vols., Berlin, 1933.

Fordham, G., *The Early History of the Central Midwives Board*, London, 1922.

Fores, S. W., *Man-Midwifery Dissected: or, the obstetric family-instructor*, London, 1793.

Foster, F., *Thoughts on the Times, but chiefly on the Profligacy of our Women, and its causes. . . . In two parts*, London, 1779.

General Lying-in Hospital, *Annual Reports*.

—— *Laws, Orders and Regulations*.

General Medical Council, *Minutes of the General Medical Council and of its Committees & branch annals*, London, 1858–

Granville, A. B., *A Report of the Practice of Midwifery at the Westminster General Dispensary, during 1818 . . .*, London, 1819.

Gregory, M. D., *A Letter to Ladies in Favour of Female Physicians*, London, 1850.

Harrison, E., M.D., *Remarks on the ineffective State of the Practice of physic in Great Britain; with proposals for its future regulation and improvement, & the resolutions of the members of the Benevolent Medical Society of Lincolnshire*, London, 1806.

Highmore, A., *Pietas Londinensis; The history, design and present state of the various public charities in and near London*, London, 1814.

Hurd-Mead, Kate Campbell, *A History of Women in Medicine from the earliest times to the beginning of the nineteenth century*, Haddam (Conn.), 1938.

Johnstone, R., M.D., *William Smellie, The Master of British Midwifery*, Edinburgh, 1952.

Kerr, J. M. M., M.D., *Maternal Mortality and Morbidity*, Edinburgh, 1933.

Kerr, J. M. M., M.D., and others, *Historical Review of British Obstetrics and Gynaecology 1800–1950*, Edinburgh, 1954.

Male Mid-Wife and the Female Doctor, The, New York, 1974.

Martineau, Harriet, 'On Female Industry', *Edinburgh Review*, April, 1859.

Mears, Martha, *The midwife's candid advice to the fair sex, or the pupil of nature: on . . . pregnancy; childbirth; the diseases incident to both*, London, 1797.

Morant, G., *Hints to Husbands: A Revelation of the Man-Midwife's Mysteries*, London, 1857.

Morland, E., *Alice and the Stork*, London, 1951.

Neff, Wanda, *Victorian Working Women*, London, 1929.

Nicholls, F., *A Petition of the Unborn Babes to the Censors of the Royal College of Physicians of London*, London, 1751.

Nightingale, Florence, *Introductory notes on lying-in institutions, together with a proposal for organizing an institution for training midwives and midwifery nurses*, London, 1871.

Nihell, Elizabeth, *A Treatise on the art of midwifery*, London, 1760.

Observations on the Impropriety of Men being Employed in the Business of Midwifery, London, 1827.

Pratt, E. A., *Pioneer Women in Victoria's Reign*, London, 1897.

Queen Charlotte's Hospital, *Annual Reports*, London.

Radcliffe, W., *The Secret Instrument*, London, 1947.

Roesslin, Eucharius, *The Byrth of Mankynde, newly translated out of Laten into Englysshe* (by R. Jonas), London, 1540.

Royal Maternity Charity, *A Plain Account of the Advantages of the Lying-in Charity for delivering poor married women at their own habitations*, London, 1767, and later editions.

St. Mary's Hospital, Manchester, *Annual Reports*.

Sermon, William, M.D., *The Ladies' Companion, or the English Midwife*, London, 1671.

Sharp, Jane, *The Midwives Book*, London, 1671.

Siebold, E. C. J. von, M.D., *Versuch einer Geschichte der Geburtshülfe, 1839–45*, 2 vols., Berlin, trans. F. S. Herrgott as *Essai d'une Histoire de l'Obstetricie*, 1891.

Stephen, Margaret, *The Domestic Midwife*, London, 1795.

Stone, Sarah, *A Complete Practice of Midwifery*, London, 1737.

Talley, W., *He- or Man-Midwifery & its Results*, London, 1863.

—— *Men in Female Attire, or the opinion of Eminent Men & Scientific Women on Delicate Subjects*, London, 1864.

Thicknesse, P., *Man-Midwifery Analysed, and the Tendency of that Practice Detected and Exposed*, London, 1764, 1765, 1790.

Thompson, Flora, *Lark Rise to Candleford*, London, 1945.

Wall, C., *The History of the Surgeons' Company, 1745–1800*, London, 1937.

Ward, E., *The London Spy Compleat, in eighteen parts*, London, 1704–6.

—— *The Whole Pleasures of Matrimony*, London, 1710.

White, C., M.D., *A Treatise on the Management of Pregnant and Lying-in Women*, London, 1773.

Willughby, P., *Observations in Midwifery. As Also the countrey Midwifes Opusculum or Vade Mecum*, H. Blenkinsop (ed.), Warwick, 1863.

Woodham-Smith, Cecil, *Florence Nightingale*, London, 1951.

NEWSPAPERS AND PERIODICALS

British Medical Journal
Englishwoman's Review
General Practitioner
Hospital with the *Hospital Nursing Mirror*
Lancet
London Medical Gazette
Medical and Physical Journal
Medical Press and Circular
Medical Times
Medical Times and Hospital Gazette
Nursing Notes
Nursing Record

Appendices

COPY OF A MIDWIFE'S LICENCE, 1686

A true Copy of my Bror.: Leo: wifes License, whose Name before
he married her was Ellen Perkins.

Henry by ye Divine permission Bishop of London, to our well
beloved in Christ Ellen Perkins the wife of Richard Perkins of ye
parrish of St. Martins in ye fields, in ye County of Middlesex, &
of our Diocess & juridiction of London, sends greeting in our
Lord God everlasting.

  Whereas by due Examination of divers honest & discreet
women, we have found you the said Ellen Perkins, apt, able, &
expert, to use & exercise the office business & function of a
Midwife, Wee therefore by our authority Ordinary & Epall, do
admit yu thereunto and give unto you full power & License to
occupie & exercise ye sd office, business & function of a Midwife
within ye City, Diocess, & jurisdiction of London with ye best
judgment, Care & diligence that yu. may or can, in that behalfe
both to poor & Rich, Streightly willing & charging you to and
for me & accomplish all things in and about the same according
to your Oath thereupon Made and Given as followeth, viz.

  Ffirst, you shall be Diligent, faithful and ready to help
every woman travilling wth. Child, as well the poor as ye Rich,
and shall not then forsake the poor woman and leave her, to go
to the Rich.

  Item, you shall neither cause nor suffer, (as far as in you
lies) any woman to Name, or put any other father to the child,
but only him who is the true father thereof indeed.

  Item, you shall not suffer any woman to pretend, feigne,
or surmise herselfe to be delivered of child, where not so indeed,
nor to claim any other womans Child for her own.

  Item, you shall not suffer any Child to be murthered,

Maimed, or otherwise hurt as much as you may, & so often as
you shall perceive any danger, or jeoperdy like to be, or ensue,
either in ye woman, or in ye Child, in such wise as yu. shall be in
doubt what may happen thereon. You shall then forthwith in due
time, send for other midwifes, & women expert in that faculty, &
use their advice and Counsel in that behalfe.

Item, you shall not in anywise use or exercise any
Manner of Witchcraft, Charm, Sorcery invocation, or other
prayers, then such as may stand with Gods Laws, and the Kings.

Item, you shall not give Counsel, nor Minister any herb,
Medicine, potion, or any other thing to any woman being wth Child,
thereby to destroy or cast out what she goeth withall before her time.

Item, You shall not enforce any woman by pains or by
any other ungodly ways, or means, to give you any more for your
pains, or Labour in bringin her to bed, then other wise she would
doe.

Item, you shall not consent, agree, give or keep Counsel
that any woman be delivered secretly of that she goeth with, but
in ye presence of two or three honest women, and that there be
always two, or three lights ready if they may be had.

Item, you shall be secret, and not open any matter
appertaining to yr. office, in ye presence of any man, unless
necessity, or very urgent occasion do constrain you so to doe.

Item, if any child be dead borne, you yourselfe shall see
it buried in such secret place, as neither Hog, Dog, nor any other
beast may come unto it, & in such sort that it be not found or
perceived as much as yu. may, and shall not suffer any such child
to be cast in the jakes, or into any other inconvenient place.

Item, if yu. shall know any Midwife using or doing any
thing contrary to any of the said premises, or any other ways
then shall be seemly & Convenient, you shall forthwith detect and
open ye same to us our Chancellour, or ye Ordinary for ye time
being.

Item, you shall use & demeane yrselfe in civil & modest
behaviour unto other women Lawfully admitted into the Roome
& office of a Midwife in all things relating thereto.

Item, you shall present to us our Chancellour or yr
ordinary for ye time being, all such women as you shall know
from time to time to occupie, or exercise the place, or function of
a Midwife within our diocess, or jurisdiction aforesaid, without
our License and jurisdiction to the same.

Item, you shall not make, or assign any Deputy, or
Deputies to exercise under you, or in your absence the office or
Room of a Midwife, but only such as yu. shall perfectly know to

be right honest & discreet women, and also apt and able having sufficient knowledge & experience to use & exercise the said place, function, and office.

Item, you shall not be privy or give consent that any priest, or other party shall in yr. absence, or in your company, or of your knowledge or sufferance, baptize any child by any Mass, latin service, or prayers, other than such as are appointed by the Laws of ye Church of England, neither shall yu. consent yt. any Child born of any woman who shall be delivered by yu, shall be carried away without being baptized in ye parish by ye Ordinary Minister where ye said Child was borne, unless it be in Case of necessity baptized privately according to ye book of common prayer, but in every such case, or cases you shall forthwith upon understanding thereof give knowledge of the same either to us the Bishop aforesaid, or our Chancellour or your Ordinary for the time being. In Witness whereof we have caused the seal of our Chancellour (which is used in this behalfe) to be set to these prets. Dated ye 14 day of August in the year 1686 and in ye Eleventh year of our Translation etc.

Derbyshire Record Office (Matlock) D.253
Memorandum Book of Titus Wheatcroft,
first Schoolmaster of Ashover (1722)

Copy of the PROSPECTUS *of the Institution recently established.*

The British Ladies' Lying-in Institution,

For Female attendance upon indigent Women at their own habitations,—for providing them with Medicines, when needful,—for supplying Women during their Confinement —and for the proper Instruction of respectable Women Midwives.

THIS Institution was established in March, 1829, by its noble Patronesses, in consequence of the reduced number and the oppressed state of respectable Midwives. It offers instruction and employment to well-educated females, and it is designed to replace the practice in the hands of that sex which nature and female decorum alike point out, while it tends to arrest the mischievous and desperate operations of violent male adventurers.

Few persons have a better claim on a humane and charitable public than the poor modest industrious Married Woman, at a period when she most requires the aid of kindness and female assistance. The pressing necessities of the labouring members of the community especially call upon those whom Providence has blest with affluence, to support this Establishment, for pre-serving female modesty, so essential to every domestic virtue, and to the general morals.

Any Lady or Gentleman becoming a Subscriber of One Guinea or more per annum, will have a right to recommend two objects for every Guinea they sub-scribe. The Subscription of Ten Guineas at one time will constitute a Donor or Life Subscriber, and will entitle her or him to recommend two patients every year.

Ladies (Subscribers or otherwise) are respectfully informed, that Donations, however small, or appropriate Linen, will be gratefully received.

Donations and Subscriptions are received by the Treasurer, Sir ANTHONY CARLISLE, 6, Langham Place; by Mr. FORES, 41, Piccadilly; and by the Secretary, Mr. T. BEALE, 10, Chapel-street, East, May Fair.

Patronesses.

Her Royal Highness the DUCHESS of KENT.
Her Grace the DUCHESS of ARGYLL,
Her Grace the DOWAGER DUCHESS of RICHMOND,
Her Grace the DUCHESS of RICHMOND,
The Right Hon. the COUNTESS of ABINGDON,
The Right Hon. the COUNTESS of BELFAST,
And other Ladies of Distinction too numerous for insertion.

President and Honorary Treasurer.

SIR ANTHONY CARLISLE, F.R.S.
Surgeon to the King, and to the Westminster Hospital.

Secretary.

Mr. T. BEALE,

Instructing and Consulting Midwives.

Mrs. BEALE,
(Professional Attendant to the original Patronesses).
Mrs. DELPINI, Mrs. DONALDSON, Mrs. GAMMAN,
Mrs. RICHARDSON, Mrs. VENN,

Attending and Practising Midwives.

Mrs. BEALE, C.M. 10, Chapel-street, May-Fair.
Mrs. BROWN, 105, Broad-wall, Blackfriars-road.
Mrs. BRIGHT, 16, George-street, Portland Chapel.
Mrs. BURTON, 3, Queen-street, Grosvenor-square.
Mrs. DELPINI, C.M. Great Newport street, St. Martin's Lane.
Mrs. DONALDSON, C.M. Gate-street, Lincoln's-inn-fields.
Mrs. DAVIS, 65, Wynatt-street, Northampton-square.
Mrs. GAMMAN, C.M. 33, East-street, Mary-le-bone.
Mrs. GODSALL, 13, Buckingham-row, Brewer's-green, Westminster.
Mrs. KELLY, 93, Devonshire-street, Mary-le-bone.
Mrs. MORTON, 4, Artillery-place, Brewer's-green, Westminster.
Mrs. MERRINGTON, 4, New-street, Brompton.
Mrs. MARSH, 10, Upper Rathbone-place.
Mrs. RICHARDSON, 52, Holborn-hill.
Mrs. VENN, C.M. 59, Wells-street, Middlesex Hospital.

Donors and Subscribers.

The COUNTESS OF MOUNTCHARLES,
The COUNTESS OF HARROWBY,
The LADY AUGUSTA CHICHESTER,
The LADY AGNES BYNG,
The LADY HENRY FITZROY,
The LADY WILLIAM GORDON,
With other Persons of Distinction too numerous for insertion.

In addition to the Subscriptions (which will be duly published) the Treasurer has to acknowledge the bene-

volent Donation of a Box, containing every requisite article for the use of a Patient and her Infant during the month of her confinement, from Her GRACE the DUCHESS of ARGYLL, and a handsome assortment of Childbed Linen from the LADY LOWE.

Since the establishment of this Institution, numerous meritorious Women have been attended by the Female Midwives, who have provided them with Linen (or a gratuity in lieu thereof), and simple medicines, such as Castor Oil, &c.

Those Ladies who may prefer the attendance of respectable females are informed, that they may be waited on at an hour's notice (in Town), by addressing a line to the Consulting Midwife, No. 10, Chapel-street, May-Fair; or if in the Country, a duly-qualified Female Midwife will be sent to reside in the family while wanted.

The President being assured from long-continued and very extensive experience, that Calomel and other mercurial drugs are highly injurious, and often prove fatal to infants; he advises the Midwives of this Institution, to resist the giving of those unnecessary poisons, and also to avoid giving Opium to Infants under any form.

THE END.

F. H. Wall, Printer, Richmond.

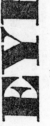

MAN-MIDWIFERY
EXPOSED!

OR,

WHAT IT IS,

AND

WHAT IT OUGHT TO BE:

Proving the practice to be injurious and disgraceful to society; the frequent cause of jealousy and disgust; and of serious mischief to delicate and modest females: with

BROAD HINTS

TO

NEW MARRIED PEOPLE,

AND

YOUNG MEN & WOMEN.

By M. ADAMS.

LONDON:

PUBLISHED BY S. W. FORES, 41, PICCADILLY; AND SOLD
BY ALL BOOKSELLERS IN THE KINGDOM.

1830.

[PRICE TWO SHILLINGS.]

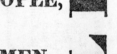

c.1870

FEMALE MEDICAL SOCIETY.

Vice-Patrons.

His Grace the DUKE OF ARGYLL, K.T.
Her Grace the DUCHESS OF ARGYLL.
ARCHBISHOP MANNING.
The BARONESS DE ROTHSCHILD.

President.

The Right Honourable the EARL of SHAFTESBURY, K.G.

General Council.

The names of the Executive Committee of the Society are marked thus *

Sir FRANCIS CROSSLEY, Bart., M.P.
Lord HOUGHTON.
Mrs. GLADSTONE.
Sir W. C. TREVELYAN, Bart.
Professor F. W. NEWMAN.
Sir JOHN BOWRING.
Miss FAITHFULL.
JOHN BAGSTER, Esq.
The Rev. JAMES MOORHOUSE, M.A.
Colonel HENRY CLINTON.
Colonel OLDFIELD.
WM. BLANCHARD JERROLD, Esq.
The Rev. W. WARD JACKSON, M.A.
WM. CRACROFT FOOKS, jun., Esq.
The Rev. JABEZ BUANE, D.D.
ARTHUR TREVELYAN, Esq., J.P.
H. OLIVER ROBINSON, Esq.

The Rev. JAMES MARTINEAU.
ISAAC WHITWELL WILSON, Esq.
W. H. D. NATION, Esq.
HENRY CARRE TUCKER, Esq., C.B.
W. S. ALDIS, Esq.
GEORGE MORANT, Esq., J.P.
*GEORGE BURNEY, Esq., Blenheim House, Bow.
*WILLIAM BARRETT, Esq., 213, High Street, Poplar.
*CHARLES HENRY ELT, Esq., 1, Noel Street, Islington.
*F. A. NEW, Esq., Oneida House, Graham Road, Dalston.
The Rev. W. D. CORKEN.
*HOLROYD CHAPLIN, Esq., 35, Blandford Square.

Educational Committee.

C. J. B. ALDIS, Esq., M.A., M.D., F.R.C.P.
WILLIAM BUCHANAN, Esq., M.D., Past Master of the Society of Apothecaries.
C. R. DRYSDALE, Esq., M.D., M.R.C.P., F.R.C.S., Physician to the Metropolitan Free Hospital, and to the North London Consumption Hospital.
DAVID HYMAN DYTE, Esq., M.R.C.S., &c.
JAMES EDMUNDS, Esq., M.D., late Senior Physician to the British Lying-in Hospital.
JOHN ELLIOTT, Esq., A.M., M.B., Physician to the Waterford Lying-in Hospital.
WILLIAM HARDWICKE, Esq., M.D., Deputy Coroner to West Middlesex.
JOHN LOCKING, Esq., M.D., Physician to the British Lying-in Hospital, and to the Islington Dispensary.
J. MACKENZIE, Esq., M.D., F.R.C.S., J.P., Provost of Inverness.
E. W. MURPHY, Esq., A.M., M.D., late Obstetric Professor at University College.
JOHN A. R. NEWLANDS, Esq., F.C.S.
GEORGE ROSS, Esq., M.D., &c.

Treasurer.—HENRY CHARLES STEPHENS, Esq., 171, Aldersgate Street, E.C.

Honorary Secretary.—JAMES EDMUNDS, Esq., M.D.

Lady Secretary.—Mrs. BLANGY.

Bankers.—The LONDON AND COUNTY BANK, 441, Oxford Street.

Temporary Offices.—4, FITZROY SQUARE, LONDON, W.

Index